Monika Jünemann • Sylvia Luetjohann

The Three Great Healing Herbs

Tea Tree, St. Johns Wort, and Black Cumin

T0149870

Monika Jünemann • Sylvia Luetjohann

The Three Great Healing Herbs

Tea Tree, St. Johns Wort, and Black Cumin

Important herbs for health and wellness
and as basics in your herbal first aid kit

Translated by Christine M. Grimm

LOTUS LIGHT
SHANGRI-LA

1st English edition 1998
© by Lotus Light Publications
    Box 325, Twin Lakes, WI 53181
The Shangri-La Series is published in cooperation
with Schneelöwe Verlagsberatung, Federal Republic of Germany
© 1997 reserved by the Windpferd Verlagsgesellschaft mbH, Aitrang
All rights reserved
Translated by Christine M. Grimm
Cover design by Kuhn Grafik, Digitales Design, Zurich, illustrations by
Elisabeth Pabst
Photographs of St. John's Wort and Black Cumin: Regina v. Hilchen
Photographs of Tea Tree: Andreas Hülsmann
Inside drawings: Elisabeth Pabst
Editing: Sylvia Luetjohann and Monika Jünemann
Composition and make-up: *panta rhei!* – MediaService Uwe Hiltmann
Production: Schneelöwe, D-87648 Aitrang

ISBN 0-914955-55-1
Library of Congress Catalogue No. 97-76422

Printed in the USA

Table of Contents

Dedication and Acknowledgements

We would like to thank the *Three Great Healers,* which supported us in compiling this book in the following ways:

❀ *St. John's Wort,* the "golden blossom", which helped us to focus the worries, which arise in writing a book, toward our inner being so that we could work with nerves strengthened by active relaxation;
❀ *Tea Tree Oil,* whose clear odor, the "spirit from the bottle", supports clear thinking and often took away our sleepiness and drove away the computer viruses;
❀ *Black Cumin,* Black Cummin or Black Caraway with many names and forms, which brought us unimagined finds in the oriental spice market and many creative ideas for new recipes and our next garden.

Our book is dedicated to these reliable helpers with thanks.

Three Superb Natural Medications

One might ask if it isn't outright arrogant to attempt to write a book about all three of these universal and superb natural medications. Not only have others posed this question, but we have asked it ourselves again and again during the research, discussions and compilation of "The three great Healers".

The volatile tea tree oil, the oil pressed from cumin at ambient temperature and the mysterious substance from St. John's wort, with its psychological effect, belong to the most popular natural medications; we want to investigate the reasons for this. Our own experiences with their use have convinced and delighted us, but we want to know why—in order to disseminate this knowledge. So we first attempted to find a common denominator for their effects and applications.

The spectrum of action by all three is extremely broad. Their main fields of application are in the treatment of infections caused by various micro-organisms and the regulation of a weakened immune system as manifested in skin and respiratory tract allergies. The effectiveness of these three medications where others fail, seems to rise from the unique synergetic composition of their components, which have no side effects.

Most of our health problems have a similar cause—infection by micro-organisms such as bacteria, viruses, parasites and increasingly even fungi. In clinical medicine, each symptom is usually treated individually; this often leads to overfilled household medicine cabinets (and a lot of poisonous refuse) as well as burdening public health services.

Real natural cures (as opposed to fashionable appearances) begin with the body as an entity and fight the actual causes of the symptoms. All three of the great cures: tea tree, St. John's wort and black cumin are natural medications capable of fighting against germs without damaging side effects and at the same time supporting the bodies own defences and potential for self healing.

Antibiotics, which are usually chemically manufactured, contain unique structural features setting them apart from the usual biological lipids and are by definition extremely reactive. They keep the symptoms in check for a while but often they have distressing side effects:

1. The mentioned side effects ("Read the information contained in the package or ...") result in other "new" complaints. Because of the toxic properties, innumerable irritations can be caused resulting in incompatibility or allergic reactions; without precautions, the toxins are often stored in the body. One unwelcome side effect is that the symbiotic coexistence of useful micro-organisms necessary for inner equilibrium is disturbed by antibiotics. For example, aggressive antibiotics disturb the lactic acid bacteria in the intestines so that the fungus (yeast fungus *candida albicans)* gets out of control.

The immune system can become weakened, overloaded, or even blocked by antibiotics. This leads to more infections since the body's natural defences are limited or lacking—so that antibiotics must be used again. The cycle runs in a circle...often the dosage must even be increased so that they work at all. This can lead to addictive type habits and dependencies on pain relievers, etc.

When an antibiotic becomes less effective or ceases to work at all, there may be another explanation:

2. Bacteria gradually develop a resistance against antibiotics so that they are figuratively "immune" against it. This is comparatively easy for the micro-organisms since chemical preparations of antibiotics usually consist of only a few substances. When bacteria are attacked by antibiotics, most of them die. Only the few resistant bacteria survive and multiply. This process of selecting individuals with an advantage is called mutation. The later generations of bacteria are more dangerous than the first.

Because they are resistant to the antibiotics they multiply more quickly and with each succeeding generation they become stronger and stronger. In order to close our vicious circle, these bacteria, which are much more dangerous than the first, must be treated with even harder and stronger antibiotics.

We can observe exactly the same mechanism in the garden: it is our experience that when plants are attacked by pests or parasites only the strongest plants survive. After an attack, a cleaver gardener, who has respect for nature, solves the problem by creating a healthy milieu in the ground which supports the needs of organisms useful for proper balance. When one uses chemicals to fight the pests, useful micro-organisms are also killed and after repeated applications, the pests become more resistant. One is forced to use more intensive poisons. The plants become weaker and their consumption less desirable because of the concentration of toxins in them ...

This leads to a comparison with our hospitals, which, in spite of all the hygienic precautions, have developed into an ideal nutrition medium for microbes that cannot be treated because they are resistant against antibiotics. Patients, who usually have weakened protection systems, are threatened by these secondary germs.

3. Although antibiotics have been used for several decades as a cure against infectious diseases, they have not eliminated them. A herb which protects us against influenza, bronchitis, or kidney and bladder infections has not yet been found. Up to now all medicaments fail in the treatment of skin diseases or the fungus mycosis. We cannot escape the thought that there might be a connection between the use of synthetically manufactured antibiotics and antiseptics and the advance of certain sickness symptoms.

Returning to our three natural healers: tea tree, St. John's wort and black cumin, we find the following advantages

❀ No irritations or toxic side effects are caused when the right dose is correctly applied.
❀ The effectiveness remains constant so that the dose must not be increased (usually the opposite is true)
❀ There may be a number of substances in the complex mixture of more than a hundred components which act to inhibit germs in subtle ways; many of the substances support the bodies own immune system.

Finally we come to the idea of testing the effectiveness of our three great healers where other medications have failed. We think of difficult infections such as fungus diseases, allergies and problems arising from a disturbed physical defence. Skin diseases have acquired a special position as "mirror" for the undisturbed equilibrium between man and the environment. The trinity formed by the immune system, the hormone system and the nervous system also responds positively to the three great healers.

Thanks to the three wonderful possibilities which nature has given us, you don't have to be confused or doubtful because you doesn't know for what or against what these great healers are best used. In addition they can be combined with each other, and even enhance each other. Despite the common bonds, closer study may reveals focal points for their application and mode of action. From experience

❀ Tea tree oil has a strongly antibacterial, anti mycotic (anti fungus) and anti viral effect when used externally, especially for skin problems and wounds, but also for infections of the mucus membrane. It is supported by
❀ St. John's wort which also has antibacterial and anti viral properties. It makes an excellent medication for external wounds but at the same time is a "balsam for inner wounds" and has the strongest mental and spiritual healing effect. Once again it is enhanced by
❀ Black cumin which can regulate too weak or too strong reactions of the immune system and appears to be pre-

destined for treating chronic, allergic and hormonal diseases.

We want, in addition, to summarize what the common features of tea tree oil, St. John's wort and black cumin are and why they shouldn't be missing from any household medicine cabinet:

❀ We aren't dealing here with medicines in the usual sense. Because the spectrum of action of these cures isn't limited to individual symptoms, they can soothe many problems. In fact, they are capable of replacing a whole row of (often) expensive medicaments.

❀ They are highly effective at a minimal dose and have no side effects so that they embody a real alternative in the treatment of a light cold or a disturbed stomach especially by people who react sensitively, tend toward allergies and/or think ecologically.

❀ Their use is many-sided since they can be used for skin and body care, cosmetics, hygiene, animal care and in the kitchen.

Since the middle of the 70's interest in alternative healing methods has risen sharply. Combined with scientific studies and modern developments directed toward the identification of the active substances, standardization, proof of their effectiveness and optimal dose, the old herb knowledge has become the modern plant and aroma therapy.

Research is important and necessary, but it is even more important that individuals assume responsibility for their own health. Use of these natural medications activates the body's own powers to protect itself. In homeopathy, which is often considered the to be the therapeutic science based on experience, not only are the symptoms of the immediate illness noted, but also portraits of the type of person that profit from the individual medications are described. Everyone finds characteristics in these portraits, which have been drawn based on the types of people which usually benefit from the respective plant medications, which mirror sides of themselves. When you elects which

medication(s) to use and concern yourself with their compatibility when used in combination, you assume part of
the responsibility for your own body and health. In this book
we do not give recommendations for a specific preparation, but attempt to compile available information so that
you are capable of making quality decisions as to the most
suited cure and the right application.

In conclusion, it should be noted that the introduction
to natural therapy is complimented by a responsible style
of life. The three great healers are not wonder tonics but
require additional thinking according to the not so simple
sentence: *prevention is better than treatment.*

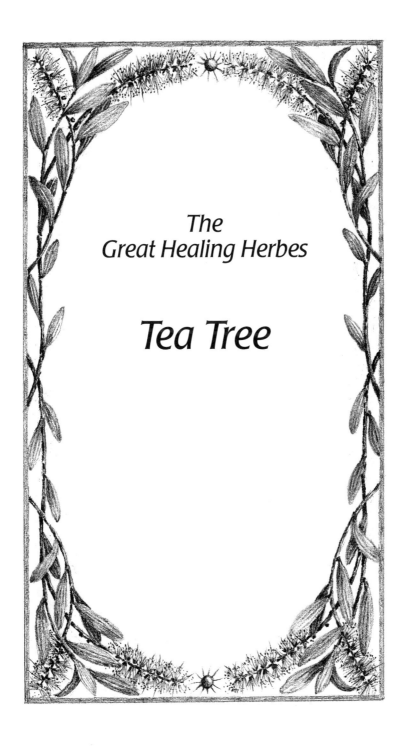

The
Great Healing Herbes

Tea Tree

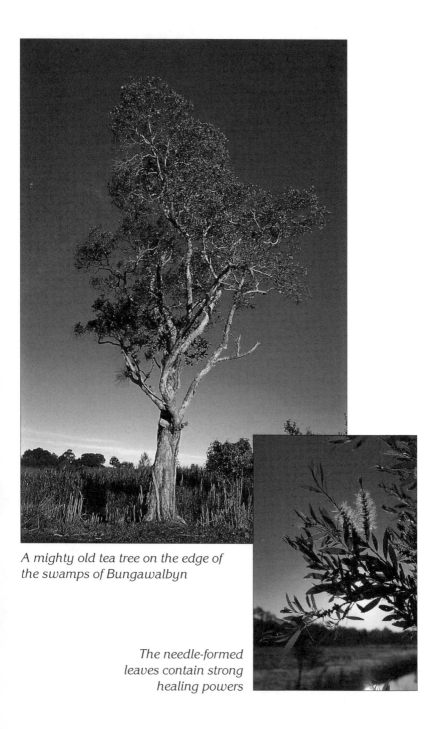

A mighty old tea tree on the edge of the swamps of Bungawalbyn

The needle-formed leaves contain strong healing powers

The very first experience with the tea tree which permanently impressed us was the decision to put a few drops of the volatile oil on the route by which ants were raiding our kitchen. All other attempts, with the exception of strong poison, had proven useless—now the success was as complete as permanent. Up until that point, the small bottle of essence, with a refreshing but strong odor and taste, had only been used sporadically for gargling. Suddenly it was the focal point of our attention; since it wasn't toxic, it obviously possessed very remarkable qualities...

In the mean time the tea tree oil, is even praised as the "green gold" of Australia; as a result of its broad spectrum of application it has become an extremely popular natural cure. The Australian tea tree or so called "Ti-Tree", which has the botanical name *Melaleuca alternifolia,* is the best known type of tea tree.

The Plant

Melaleuca alternifolia belongs to the family of myrtle plants (*Myrtaceae)* together with eucalyptus, cajeput, common myrtle, and the two other tea trees of the Type Leptospermum, red manuka and white manuka, which will be discussed later.

The plant is a native of the subtropical bush land of New South Wales on the eastern coast of Australia. The best quality tea tree oil comes from the humid and swampy areas of Bungawalbyn in northern New South Wales. There are many other species of tea trees—in Australia there are an estimated 300 species. They are also found in South Africa, India, and Malaysia.

The bush-like trees which remain green all year, are cultivated on large plantations where they reach a height of six feet. Under natural conditions, they reach a height of up to twenty four feet. They have narrow, needle shaped leaves similar to cypresses; their strongly fragrant white flowers remind one of the aroma of eucalyptus oil.

The white settlers on the northern coast of New South Wales considered the tea tree as a "plague" because it hindered them from drying out the swamps in order to cultivate "useful plants". The tea tree, like the rest of its family, is extremely tough; in particular it has very persevering, deep roots. If they are not all removed when it is cut, new sprouts quickly appear. It has developed an effective protection against its natural enemies, including insects, bacteria, viruses and fungi. The volatile oil in its leaves has made it an old healing and spice plant.

The Volatile Oil from the Tea Tree

Many volatile oils have healing and protective characteristics. The tea tree belongs to the plants which are not only able to protect themselves against fungi, bacteria and other parasites, but also man from the same plagues (as well as from allergies and toxins). As the aroma therapist Robert Tisserand explained: oil from the tea tree "is one of the most effective and most compatible volatile oils with anti microbial characteristics.

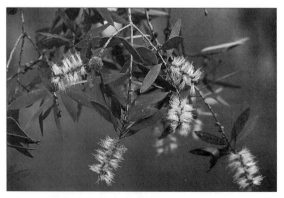

The white flowers release a strong aromatic fragrance

18

The Aborigines, the original inhabitants of Australia, naturally knew about the antiseptic effect with wounds—even the white settlers were forced to recognize this once they acquired injuries by clearing away the tea trees. The pressed flowers mixed with warm clay, can be applied as a compression which disinfects and heals wounds.

The Fascinating Story of Discovery

The popular English name "tea tree" goes back to Captain James Cook, the famous Englishman who sailed around the world in search of "*Terra australis*". When he landed in 1770 at Botany Bay on the north-eastern coast of Australia, his crew made a tea from the leaves of the trees which grew there. It was a refreshing "tea substitute". Probably it raised their spirits; regarding possible healing effects, however, can only be speculated. Sir Joseph Banks, the botanist of this expedition, took two samples of the sticky leaves back to England to study, but the medical value of the tea was apparently not discovered. Not until 150 years later was the strong anti septic and bacterial effect established.

The Ancient Knowledge of the Aborigines

The oil was known to the Aborigines, particularly the Bundjalung tribe, for hundreds or thousands of years. Because of its exceptional antiseptic properties, it was useful for the treatment of wounds, cuts, burns, sunburn, skin infections, furuncles and blisters. Broken leaves were laid on wounds or the afflicted areas and covered with a warm mud. The Bundjalung also used the healing powers of the tea tree for mouth sores, toothaches, sore throats and colds. By rubbing various types of leaves (which are referred to today as "chemical types"), they were able to determine the best application. When there was a strong eucalyptus fragrance, indicating a high cineol content, the volatile active component helped by respiratory illness. When there was a weaker fragrance, indicating a lower cineol content and higher terpinenol-(4) content, a particularly antiseptic (germ killing) effect was present.

The First Rediscovery of Tea Tree Oil

From 1923 to 1925, the chemist Arthur Penfold carried out a study on *Melaleuca alternifolia* for the government in Australia. In 1925 he was able to show that an antiseptic effect which was 11 – 13 times stronger than phenol, one of the chemicals which was used at that time. The tea tree oil dissolved blisters and even eliminated infection from dirty wounds. An early study also proved the astonishing property that the presence of blood, pus or other organic substances actually increased its antiseptic effect by 10 – 12%. Yet it was neither toxic nor irritating, In contrast, other known antiseptics attack the tissue as well as bacteria. With the outbreak of the second world war, the advantages of tea tree oil made it a "military raw material" needed in the first aid kits of the army and marines.

During the course of the war, tea tree oil was forgotten for a few decades because scientists were more interested in synthetically manufactured medicines like the antibiotics used today, particularly penicillin. This "wonder remedy" had the advantage that it could be chemically synthesized in every desired quantity.

The Second Rediscovery of Tea Tree Oil

In 1976 an unconventional Australian family conceived the plan of creating a tea tree farm in Bungawalbyn in order to produce high quality tea tree oil. This plan was based on personal experience with the volatile oil in the treatment of fungus under toenails. Their tiny plantation was an enormous success in a few natural food stores and alternative markets. The following figures establish the victory of this "help from the bottle":

yearly production 1985 = about 10 tons
yearly market 1992 = about 700 tons

It is easy to see that the still growing needs could scarcely be met by the swamp area of New South Wales.

Harvest of Tea Tree Leaves

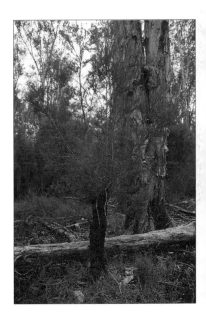

Originally the leaves were harvested from the swamps by hand. With a light but sharp knife, the harvesters made their way through the bush, cut the shoots from the trunk and scraped the leaves from the branches and twigs. The leaves and twigs were carried in jute sacks to the distillery oven. An experienced harvester could gather a ton of tea tree leaves in one day, from which ten quarts of volatile oil could be obtained.

As difficult as this method may have been, it had the advantage that no trees hat to be replanted. Apparently stimulated by the pruning, the leaves grew back on their own at an astonishing rate. The trees in Bungawalbyn that have been harvested on a regular basis since 1925 are among the strongest and produce an oil of the highest quality. Even up until 1988, the leaves of the tea trees were gathered in this way by individual harvesters.

Modern Plantations

Soon the constantly increasing demands for tea tree oil could not be filled by the limited region in New South Wales. Tea trees require swamps for optimal development, but

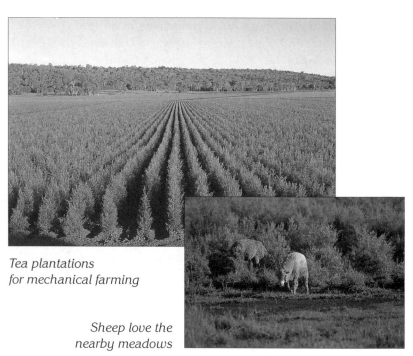

*Tea plantations
for mechanical farming*

*Sheep love the
nearby meadows*

they must not necessarily be in the deep Australian bush; they can also lie in somewhat more accessible humid areas. Rich soils make it possible for them to grow quickly. For plantation cultivation, trees are selected whose quality of oil is not subject to large variations. Smaller, bushy trees are planted so that harvesting is easier. In order to combine an optimal harvest with the principles of ecological equilibrium, the tea-tree farmer has been forced to carry out a lot of experimentation.

Steam—the Magic of Distillation

Tea leaves and twigs are usually dumped into a large kettle of water which is slowly heated with a wood fire. As the temperature rises, the veins of the leaves break open and the contents from hundreds of tiny "pockets" or vesicles are released. These large molecules hydrolyze (react with water) and are borne by steam into the gaseous phase. When passed through a condenser (tube cooled with water), the oil becomes liquid. Since it floats on the top of water it can be simply removed. Then it is filtered and filled into small bottles. Each batch of tea tree oil is chemically analyzed since oil from trees growing wildly in the bush always have varying quality. The condensed fragrant water yields the tea tree hydrolyzate, which is used primarily in skin care.

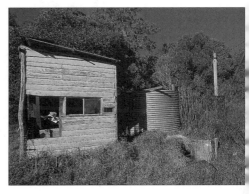

One needs little more than a kettle and fire for the traditional distillation

Active Ingredients of Tea Tree Oil

The essence of the tea tree varies from almost colorless to a pale lemon yellow and has an extremely characteristic odor—very spicy and strong, almost "medical"; that of the wild trees is the strongest. It is similar to that of eucalyptus or camphor or nutmeg. The literature often lists 48 different components, but according to more recent research there are about 100. The larger number apparently arises from a longer distillation time (up to four hours). From this multiplicity and synergetic co-operation, the optimal healing effect of the tea tree oil arises—and at the same time the suspected difficulty of Bacteria & Company to make themselves immune against it ...

The contents include monoterpenols, monoterpenes such as pinene, alpha and gamma terpinene and p-cymene, cineole, sesquiterpenes and sesquiterpene alcohols. The quality depends primarily on the content of 1,8 cineole and terpinenol-(4).

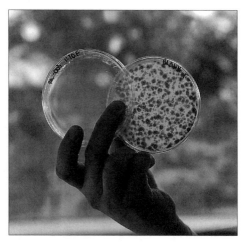

*The strong anti bacterial effect
can be seen experimentally*

Cineole versus Terpinenol-(4)

Arthur Penfold determined together with other researchers, that the essence of various tea trees was subject to large variations. Trees of the same botanical origin could produce oil of totally different composition. Depending on the dominance of one particular substance, various *chemical types* were distinguished, from which the degree of effectiveness in various applications depends.

Tea tree oil can contain a considerable amount of terpinenol-(4) (up to 45%) and little cineole, as indicated by an odor similar to nutmeg. The other possibility is a high

24

cineole content (varies between 2 – 65%) so that it can be compared with eucalyptus oil which is rich in cineole; this variation can be recognized by a camphor fragrance. Cineole heals colds but irritates the mucous membrane and burns the skin so that it should not be used for infections or wounds at higher concentrations.

In contrast, an oil whose content of terpinenol-(4) is too low, is found to be less effective medically than might be expected since terpinenol-(4) has strong antibacterial properties, eliminates poisons and strengthens the immune system, increases the body's production of hormones and has a particularly regenerative healing effect. According to the official criteria, the concentration of terpinenol-4 should be at least 30%, while cineole must lie under 15%. The "Rolls Royce" of tea tree oils even has a terpinenol-(4) content of 40% or more and a cineole content of less than 4%.

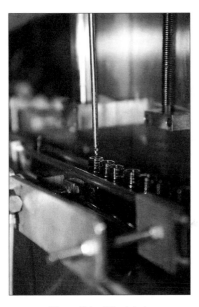

The oil is filled into 10 ml bottles

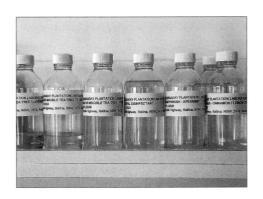

The contents must be constantly controlled

25

Just Clever Product-Marketing?

A critical comment should be made here with respect to a phenomenon that might be an expression of clever "product marketing": This has to do with the requirements for terpinenol-(4) and 1,8-cineole.

Commercially, other *melaleuca* types (such as *Melaleuca linarifolia* or *M. dissitiflora*) are sold as "tea tree oil", when they meet the standards for terpinenol-(4) and cineole. Since the range allowed is extremely broad, there is the danger that the oil is often "cut" according to these restrictions. If the cineole content is lowered and the terpinenol-(4) content raised by further mixing, the oil looses its natural total constitution, and possibly a part of its natural healing power.

An additional consequence of this "product marketing" is that tea tree oil which does not come from a controlled biological culture, may stem from plants whose development has been strongly manipulated. Even at a cineole content under 3.5% and a terpinenol-(4) over 35%, skin irritations can be observed. The so-called "cosmetic" quality level C should in no case be used without dilution.

We would like to emphasize in this connection that the natural matrix is important since individual components are not used alone. Cineole is one of the most commonly occurring oxygen containing components in most volatile oils and a particularly important active component in the entire plant family of myrtle. When taken internally, cineole dissolves slime and cramps as well as killing germs. Only at an extremely high dose, does it become toxic, paralyzing the nervous system, reducing the blood pressure, frequency of breathing and body temperature. In her book "Australian Tea Tree Oil Guide—First Aid Kit in a Bottle", Cynthia Olsen reports several cases in which children accidentally drank 25 ml (about an eighth of a cup) of tea tree oil and as a consequence were only sleepy for 24 hours and had light diarrhoea.

Quality is Important

Since inexpensive oils are often diluted or even cut so that they are "identical with natural oils", it is recommended that one buy tea tree oil in a health food store or drug store and to watch for the following:

- ❀ 100% volatile oil
- ❀ From wild growth, controlled biological cultivation or (when conventional cultivation) controlled for residue
- ❀ Land of origin
- ❀ Listing of the English (or German) and Latein botanical plant names.

A definite odor like camphor and a sweet aroma are probably an indication of a high cineole content. To test the purity, let a drop of tea tree oil fall onto a filter paper. By a pure volatile oil, no fat spot remains after a while—otherwise the plant oil has been extended. Synthetically manufactured oils can be made to smell like the natural oil, but it would be practically impossible to synthesize an oil with the same healing effect.

Tea Tree Oil–the Secret of its Healing Power

According to Robert Tisserand, tea tree oil belongs to the most exciting re-discovered ethereal oils of the last years and plays an important role in aroma therapy.

Plant therapy or the study of the healing power of plants deals with the entire plant, while aroma therapy uses the volatile oil obtained by distillation of the plant components. Tea tree oil is an excellent remedy against all types of infectious processes such as bronchitis, sinusitis, tooth abscesses and gum infections, contageous, viral and parasite intestinal infections as well as fungus infections. The broad spectrum of application results from its antiseptic (anti bacterial), anti viral and fungus properties and—as protection—the stimulation of the immune system, so that it can act more effectively against microbes and germs.

❀ Because of the *antiseptic* effect against bacteria, tea tree oil is suitable for the treatment of wounds, cuts, burns, skin problems, infections of the respiratory path (bronchitis, sinusitis) and the urinary tract (bladder and vagina infections).

❀ Because of the *anti viral* effect it can be used for colds, numerous infection diseases, Herpes, shingles, and even chickenpox and German measles. Viruses are extremely difficult to treat since they penetrate into cells and are much more difficult for the immune system to recognize and fight than bacteria. Almost all antibiotics are useless against them.

❀ As a result of its *fungicide* effect, tea tree oil fights fungal infections such as *candida albicans* (in the intestine or vagina) as well as skin and foot fungi and nail mycoses.

In addition tea tree oil is

❀ generally analgesic, anti inflamatory, and supports healing of wounds and scars

❀ decongestive and soothing for throat, breast, and the respiratory pathways

❀ effective against parasites and insects.

The French aroma therapist Rodolphe Balz* even said it "protects against radiation damage" such as burns from radiation therapy. Perhaps further research will find the most effective chemical types of tea tree oil for the various areas of application.

---

* "The Healing Power of Essential Oils", Lotus Light Publications, Twin Lakes 1996

The Effect on the Immune System

Tea tree oil can be used as a general prophylactic, to treat lingering, chronic sicknesses (for example, gland fever, hepatitis, chronic-exhaustion-syndrome; tests with aids have begun) as well as raising the body's defences before an operation.

Three different types of cell groups, the phagocytes, the T-cells and the B-cells, which are formed from white blood cells in the bone marrow or the thymus, protect the body against infections. When this protection system is damaged or weakened, the body becomes more susceptible to germs. Volatile oils enhance the production of antitoxins and the number of white blood cells increases—an effect which is therapeutically termed "healing leucocytosis".

The immune system is supported by other body functions, especially the lymph system and the nervous system. Recent research has also shown that a sluggish immune system can be caused in part by emotional and psychological factors. Tea tree oil can do a lot here by fighting pathogenic materials, arousing the organs and cells involved, as well as strengthening the immune system. Through its urine stimulating and anti toxic effect in bladder infections, poisonous substances are eliminated by the kidneys which could otherwise get into the blood stream.

The Mental/Spiritual Effect

*Fragrances reach areas of the brain which are not subject to consciousness; their perception influences our psyche and changes our inclinations (*Marguerite Maury)

Through the connections between the sense of smell, the brain and the nervous system, there is a connection between sense of smell and thoughts, feelings and moods.

Volatile oils can cause the release of hormones and substances with a neurochemically active effect.

The psychic effects of tea tree oil can be drawn from the strong life force in the tea tree in its natural surroundings and from its enormous resistance against damaging influences: it is practically impossible to get rid of it. When one considers under what difficult environmental conditions the tea tree prevails, one can appreciate what powers of resistance it has developed and can give in concentrated form to mankind.

Tea tree oil is a real tonic for the circulatory system and nerves and also helps by general and nervous asthenia as a result of its high content of monoterpenes. For this purpose, one either uses it for a foot or stomach massage or vaporizes it in an aroma lamp.

Tea Tree Oil in the Aroma Lamp

The active substances of a volatile oil are taken up by the nose, the respiratory pathway and the lungs as well as over the skin and mucous membrane. This happens when the oil components are added to the room's atmosphere by vaporizing the oil together with water in an aroma lamp. Mental reactions are caused by the end effect of these substances on the brain; in the same way, an effect on the hormone household takes place. After about half an hour, the body is penetrated by the fine material vibrations of the ethereal oil and enriched by their particularly energetic power.

Tea tree oil is as clear and pure as its aroma and supports clear, logical thoughts and actions. This odor has a refreshing and strengthening effect, is activating but not relaxing like lavender, East Indian Geranium *(Cymbopogon martinti)*, or all citric oils. Lavender, through its high content of esters (40 – 50%), has a very relaxing mental effect and is an ideal addition to the concentrated power of the tea tree. Often tension and a lack of relaxation are the basis of sickness. Lavender in combination with tea tree oil even helps against sleep disturbances (together with St. John's wort as a massage). In this case the strong medicinal character is softened by the pleasant mixture of fragrances.

By sensitive, slightly fearful persons, the tea tree oil is stabilizing and dissolves fears. Relaxation is enhanced by mixing with lavender and East Indian Geranium *(Cymbopogonin martinti)* in equal portions; one has more self confidence and through this more energy and stamina.

When self confidence is strengthened, one has no problems with the world and co-inhabitants. For this, a fragrant mixture of tea tree, marjoram, rosewood or tea tree, lemon and mimosa is recommended.

Important:
*For the use of tea tree oil in water, for example by rinses and baths, one needs an **emulsifier**, in order to distribute it throughout the water in the form of an emulsion by vigorous mixing or shaking. Lukewarm warm milk or cream (not over 45 degrees Fahrenheit) is recommended.*

The Best Dose

Tea tree oil with its relatively low cineole content is much more compatible than eucalyptus oil (cineole is sometimes called "eucalyptus oil"). However, one is advised to avoid large quantities and prolonged internal use of tea tree oil. In the case of children, who accidentally drank 25 ml (about an eighth of a cup) of undiluted oil, only sleepiness and diarrhoea occurred; the symptoms disappeared after one day. *Candida* and aids patients who took 60 drops over several months and the therapist who took 120 drops daily for three months had no side effects. However, we do not recommend such a high dosage!

A number of publications generally advise against the internal use of tea tree oil. It is recommended only in exceptional cases under medical supervision and for a maximum of 14 days. We mix one drop with some honey, kept it in the mouth for a few minutes and then swallow it. In this manner the active ingredients can easily be taken up by the mucous membranes of the stomach and intestinal tract.

Even when application is made *externally*, one is again and again advised to caution—because of the possibility of low concentration(s) of potentially toxic substance(s) and a too concentrated cineole content which can lead to allergic reactions of the skin and mucous membrane. It is best to make a test with the undiluted oil on the back of the wrist and to watch for a possible reaction for an hour. In such cases, tea tree oil should only be applied after dilution with water or a skin oil. One can also obtain a mixture diluted with water and containing 15% essence commercially; in this dose it is also still very effective. Originally in Australia, the pure essence (Ti-Trol) was used on closed skin areas while the dilute water solution (Melasol) was used for injured skin, for infected, open tissue and in th inner body cavities.

Tea tree oil—one of the most popular all-round Remedies

The components of the tea tree are not only available as a pure (or diluted with water) ethereal oil or the hydrolyzate from the distillation, but also, in the meantime, as a component of numerous products available in the natural food stores, on the shelves of supermarkets, and in catalogues. Tea tree oil is valued by natural therapists, dentists, massagists and chiropractors, and is used, for example, in Swiss hospitals. Through its many sided, useful antiseptic capabilities, it has become a not so easy to replace medication at home and in first aid kits.

It has an effect which is many times stronger than other disinfectants on the market. In addition to its healing abilities, its anti microbial and anti toxic properties are particularly useful; for example, by an otherwise deadly bite of the *Antrax robustus* spider (found only in New South Wales but comparable with the "black widow").

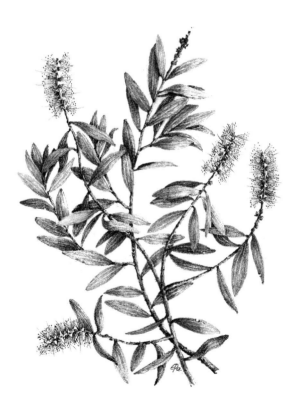

The tea tree twigs in bloom

THE BEST APPLICATIONS FOR TEA TREE OIL

Precise directions for the use and recipes can be found in the Appendix "Applications from A – Z."

Tea tree oil as Antiseptic—as an example, the Skin

The skin is the largest and most sensitive organ in our body. At the same time it forms the border to the outside world, transferring messages from the outer world. Numerous nerve endings and detective bodies record and transfer the signals and stimulations from outside to the brain. There is such a close connection between the skin and our psyche through the transmitters and hormones, that it is said to be a "mirror of the soul". This connection is obvious through expressions like "jump out of his skin", "to get under the skin" or "to feel good in your skin" because something "doesn't itch".

Our skin is closely connected with the immune system; its cells have the ability to form and mobilize substances which fight infections. Skin problems often express a weak immune system together with a disturbed psychic equilibrium. Inner conflicts force their way outside and form acne, more or less allergic skin irritations, dandruff flakes or *neurodermitis.*

Psoriasis (dandruff flakes) are caused by the disturbed function of the skin enzyme, an increased flaking of the skin cells and a broadening of the capillaries. Stress as well as mental and emotional burdens—together with environmental influences, food allergies and lack of vitamins—are often held responsible alone or in combination with other factors.

The Effect of Tea Tree Oil on the Skin

The spectrum of application of tea tree oil in connection with the skin is very large. We read from an enthusiastic user:

I always put tea tree oil on concussions or burns. The pain decreases, no blisters are formed and no scars remain... I even put tea tree oil on cuts or insect bites as well as muscle pains. A reduction of pain can be felt immediately....
(Veronica M., 47 years)

Can one believe it? Mistletoe, called *Uchelwydd* or "Heal All", that was worn by the Druids, must fear the loss of its unchallenged position. But the contents of and the way tea tree oil works have been scientifically studied and practically tested.
It works
❀ antiseptically
❀ cleansing and disinfecting.

It has the properties of
❀ penetrating deeply into the pores and tissue
❀ doesn't irritate the skin and
❀ doesn't damage the tissue cells.

In addition it has
❀ an almost neutral pH value
❀ a fresh odor
❀ good grooming characteristics

In comparison with other disinfecting medications, tee tree oil is very effective and compatible as a result of its low cineole content. Healthy tissue is handled with care and the skin isn't dried out. Irritations don't occur—only with the eyes is the greatest precaution recommended. Tea tree oil has the ability to penetrate into deeper lying tissues where it can dissolve pus focal points and has an anti inflammatory effect. It attacks the center of infections and destroys the accumulated pus like a solvent.

With abscesses and boils, the fast healing of the pus focal points is explained by the germ killing effect on the bacteria *Staphylococcus aureus.* By applying the tea tree oil (either pure or in a diluted emulsion), operations on furuncle can usually be avoided.

With acne and seborrhoea, dermatitis, skin rashes and flakes, psoriasis, neurodermitis, allergic and other itching skin irritations, even by chickenpox (and naturally also by insect bites see below) the often unbearable itching is lessened by tea tree oil and the healing process encouraged. One should try it out on a small area before applying it to a large area; if it reacts in an allergic manner, it should be diluted. One can also put a few drops of tea tree oil in warm water or in your own skin care products.

In stores one can also find tea tree soap and non fat antiseptic skin creams or moisture lotions. Often warts disappear, especially the annoying ingrown warts on the feet, after regular application—and a lot of patience.

Tea tree oil can also be used against Herpes, an infectious blister rash which spreads over the entire body and can be caught by others. It is caused by a virus. Most antiseptic medications are too sharp and irritate the sensitive skin even more. Apply tea tree oil directly; it dries the infection center out and prevents its spread and the formation of new blisters and, thereby, supports the healing process. Diluted tea tree oil can also be applied with the necessary care together with a doctor's treatment, for example as an addition to the bath, by genital Herpes and the related shingles.

The Treatment of Wounds

By scrapes, cuts, contusions, etc. tea tree oil has a gentle disinfectant effect, kills dangerous bacteria and accelerates healing. As a result of the already mentioned ability to penetrate into deep tissue and dissolve the abscess, the surface of infected wounds is cleaned so that the germ killing effect of tea tree oil can work better. Even deeper sitting particles of dirt are loosened and can be pushed away. Furthermore, tea tree oil increases blood circulation through the tiny capillaries bringing oxygen, nutrients and infection inhibiting white blood cells.

In Australia, a geriatric study was carried out on effects of tea tree oil on the legs of older patients with diabetics or other sicknesses associated with ageing. Treatment made dry skin areas softer and skin tears healed without scars establishing the bactericide and repair properties of the oil contents. The skin of older people is considerably more sensitive than that of younger people and regenerates much more slowly. Burns and sunburn can also be treated with tea tree oil directly or with an antiseptic fat free tea tree cream. This softens the pain, prevents blisters from forming and protects from further infection. By large surface areas, compressions can be applied. For this type of application, tea tree essence should be diluted with water and not with an oil: 5 ml tea tree oil (eventually with lavender oil) in 1 quart of water (0.5%).

Tea Tree Oil for Fungus Infections

Many fungi are useful for man, live in a type of "symbiosis" with him, and maintain the balance between his organism and uncountable micro-organisms. Under certain conditions, however, they can gain the upper hand, spread throughout the entire body, and weaken the immune system. Pathogenic yeasts, especially *Candida albicans,* attack the skin, mucous membrane (vagina), the skin under the nails, and can even attack the inner organs. These feared yeast fungi are extremely infectious and necessitate a high geared antiseptic treatment, without irritating the infected skin or the mucous membrane. In contrast to most other ethereal oils, tee tree oil can be used in the right dilution even in the genital area.

As a fungicide for external use, tea tree oil has the following advantages:

❀ It is skin compatible and almost never irritates, even diluted it is very effective.

❀ By penetrating deep into the tissue and mucous membrane, it fights the root of the problem.

❀ It is generally antiseptic—a "broad-band-medication"

❀ Through its numerous, many-sided, active components, it assists in the body's fight on a number of levels making it difficult for even adaptable germs.

❀ It has no side effects.

With athlete's foot, tea tree oil has proven to be very effective—undiluted as well as mixed with skin-oil or diluted with water to a 40% solution. It is necessary to apply it to the affected area regularly, twice daily over an extended time period. By *nail Mycoses* and fungus nail infection, one softens the nail for 5 minutes twice daily and then massages the surrounding area. (Incidentally, tea tree oil also helps to alleviate other foot problems such as foot perspiration, toe calluses, etc.)

From *Candida* fungus infection there is itching, infection and a strong white excretion. Vaginal infections can also be caused by *trichomonaden* (single celled parasites) or bacteria; the symptoms are very similar. Application of tea tree oil (for vagina wash or in a bath) as a broad-band-medicament eliminates the complications of a "wrong diagnosis"!

After completing two sets of experiments on yeast fungus infection (an attack of the vagina by *Candida albicans*) and chronic cystitis (bladder infection), the French Professor for Plant Therapy Paul Belaiche reported:

We are very happy with the results...the ethereal oil of the Malaleuca has its place among the most important ethereal oils and has established itself as a first class, aroma therapy weapon in the fight against germs and fungus afflictions.

Tea Tree Oil for Skin and Body Care

Through its extraordinary antiseptic properties, skin creams and other body care products are capable of inhibiting bacteria when only 2% tea tree oil is added. Soaps, shampoos, shower gels and lotions with tea tree oil have a spicy fresh fragrance. The components of the oil penetrate deep into the skin (increasing the blood flow with subsequent oxygen enrichment) and support regeneration of the skin damaged by environmental influences (strong sun, dryness) or skin diseases (acne, fungus germs). The oil is very compatible and causes—with the exception of the eyes—no irritation, but has a decided soothing effect on irritated skin. Even the tea tree water which collects the highly effective water soluble components, referred to as hydrolyzate, is good for cleansing the skin.

A few drops of tea tree oil can easily be mixed into hair shampoos, shower gels, liquid soap, skin oil etc. A broad selection of skin-care products is available.

Tea tree soap is very good for the skin and for skin problems such as eczema, rash and fungus infection. As a result of its high boiling point, the essence does not loose its healing properties when mixed with soap. Although it isn't irritating, it has a stronger germ-killing effect than germ-killing soaps containing phenol. Shower gels with tea tree oil are also available.

Tea tree skin creams made with a water base have about 5% tea tree oil. Direct application to all skin irritations has a soft, soothing, antiseptic effect.

Tea tree hair shampoo (with 2% tea tree oil) is very compatible with sensitive skin tending toward eczema, as well as for dandruff, fatty hair, and milk-scall (crusta lactea in babies). It strengthens the hair and supports hair growth. *Before* washing the hair, one can massage 5 drops of pure tea tree essence into the scalp and let it work for 5 minutes.

Teeth and Mouth Hygiene

Tea tree toothpaste is commercially available and is very effective in preventing cavities and inhibiting plaque forming bacteria which cause gingivitis. One can rub the gums directly with tea tree oil or put a few drops in the gargle water—with broad band effect as suggested in the following report:

I put 1 drop of tea tree oil in the toothpaste (one can also drop it directly onto the toothbrush to disinfect it) when I brush my teeth.. When I have a sore throat, I gargle several times a day with 3 – 5 drops of tea tree oil in two mouthfuls of warm water. This also helps against gum bleeding. When I have a gum infection, I rub tea tree oil directly on the gum. Improvement can be felt immediately.
(Sylvia M., 22 years)

Finally *tea tree lipstick* should be mentioned, it requires getting used to because of its strong taste, but soon one doesn't want to be without it by every wind and weather. It not only helps dry, cracked lips under extreme weather conditions, but also protects those who tend toward infection, blisters and even Herpes.

Tea Tree Oil in Baby Care

Tea tree oil should never be used undiluted here.

Diaper rash can be treated with a dilute and warm solution of oil or with a mild tea tree lotion. As an additional precaution, the diapers can be softened in a solution of 4 quarts of water with 20 drops of tea tree oil. Often the fungus *Candida albicans* occurs together with diaper rash usually as a mouth infection. A very dilute (because of the taste) solution can be dabbed on it.

By *milk-scall* on the scalp, massage a mixture of 5 drops of tea tree oil and 50 drops of a soft, skin oil (almond pressed at ambient temperature) into the scalp. Let it work for a few minutes and rinse well. Tea tree shampoo can also be used if care is taken.

Tea Tree Oil at Home

Tea tree oil is very suitable for disinfecting rooms, especially from patients. For this purpose, a number of varieties with high cineole content are available. This is a good substitute for strong chemicals and, in addition, eliminates odors. For basic cleaning, even for house dust mites, 20 – 40 drops in the wash water keeps insects away. One can achieve the same effect by vaporizing tea tree oil in the aroma lamp. Many people prefer a mixture with lavender and lemon oil to the pure oil.

Insects and Insect Bites

A completely natural means of defence, tea tree oil drives insects away without necessarily killing them. The already mentioned ant pathway, which wound through a kitchen window in our old house, was so thoroughly stopped that in the following years, just placing the bottle in the window was enough to keep the uninvited gusts away.

When one rubs tea tree oil into the skin, flies, mosquitoes and other insects are repelled. If one is bitten, one can apply tea tree oil directly to the bite. Itching is reduced and a possible infection prevented (which can happen very quickly by scratching—not only by children!) Tea tree oil can be used alone or mixed with 5 drops of red manuka and 10 drops of lavender.

The tea tree harvesters were the first to use the essence for repelling insects (including ticks) as well as leeches. When they cut their way through the Australian Bush, they sprayed their socks with it. If a drop of tea tree oil is placed on a tick, it dies immediately and can be easily removed with a pair of tweezers; at the same time the bite is disinfected. For flee, bee and wasp bites, tea tree oil mixed with some skin oil can work wonders.

Tea Tree Oil in Animal Care

The experiences so far reported can be directly applied to pets: The pure oil can be massaged into wounds and injuries, areas frequently scratched and eczema. For small animals it should be mixed with a carrier oil.

For flees, one mixes a few drops of tea tree oil in the normal shampoo or sprays the fur with a diluted oil. Especially with cats, one should use very little tea tree oil diluted with water or oil.

For ticks, it is recommended that a few drops of tea tree oil be placed directly on the pest, wait a little and then turn the tick with tweezers. A few drops of tea tree oil on the area prevents infection and accelerates the healing process.

THE NEW ZEALAND TEA TREES RED MANUKA AND WHITE MANUKA

Two ethereal oils which are less well known and still difficult to obtain, come from tea trees in New Zealand: red and white manuka. Both belong to the myrtle plants but are not the Melaleuca type like the Australian tea tree but belong to the *Leptospermum* genus. They are found on the northern islands of New Zealand, for example the peninsula Coromandel, and thrive in the marshes as well as the snow capped mountain peaks.

They have developed a particularly strong protection system against the forces of nature (and also man), against insects, viruses and fungi, especially in the ethereal oil of the many small glands on the under side of every leaf. These have a high content of *leptospermone*—a natural anti bacterial agent which is contained in the ethereal oil as well as in red manuka honey. It has a triketone cyclohexyl core and its structure is comparable with the synthetically manufactured valone, an anti worm agent, which also has anti bacterial properties. However, leptospermone is considerably more effective.

The History of the (possible) Discovery

Farmers raising red and white manuka trees in New Zealand today claim the name "tea tree", which Captain James Cook and his botanist Sir Joseph Banks gave to the tree providing a spicy tasting and refreshing tea, really belongs to the red manuka tea tree. Supposedly James Cook also used red manuka leaves as a component for making beer and his crew chewed red manuka seeds against diarrhoea—a custom, which has persisted until today.

Which plant is the "real" tea tree? Our research has shown that Captain Cook apparently discovered red manuka during his second world trip (1772 – 1775) as he wrote in his book which was published in 1777. Toward the end of the 18th century, the German botanists note two forms of Cook's "tea tree"—from the genus *Melaleuca and Leptospermum.*

Red Manuka

We first heard of red manuka in the form of an amber colored honey from natural food store owners. Apart from the precious aroma, which is reminiscent of the best types of southern, European, moor honey or Macchia honey, its wonderful effects on health and the strengthening of the immune system have been praised. In spite of its strong taste, no one has had the idea to eat crystalized tea tree oil...

The Plant

The botanical name of the red manuka tree is *Leptospermum scoparium.* It is also usually called "tea tree" and "red manuka". *Manuka* is the name given it by the Maoris, who used it traditionally to treat diarrhoea and wounds. The brew from its leaves was also used for urinary tract infections and colds with fever.

On the northern islands of New Zealand, red manuka is, the most widespread plant. The fast growing and especially resistant trees are planted for regeneration of large areas, which the white settlers previously made "useful" by burning. They can reach twenty four feet, have small pointed, almost spiny leaves and many white to rose colored, very fragrant flowers.

The Volatile Oil

The yellow, viscose oil is obtained by steam distillation. There is not very much red manuka oil because the distillation yield is so limited: 1 quart of oil from 3 tones of green leaves. Since 1993, there is a mixture with oil from white manuka leaves which is labeled (New Zealand's) "tea tree oil". Red and white manuka oils are considered to be a particularly effective biological broad band medication.

Composition

Although red manuka oil, like the Australian melaleuca tea tree oil, has a strong anti bacterial and germ killing effect, it differs in its chemical composition: it has a large amount of the particularly soothing triketone cyclohexyl ring derivatives (for example, leptospermone) and of sesquiterpenes (such as cadinene), which are similar to those in cedar wood. For this reason it is especially suited for the skin and mucous membrane. Its anti mycotic effect (for example by *Candida*) is even stronger than that of tea tree oil. But here it is important to test it before using without dilution!

Special Applications

Red manuka is, like all tea tree types, very robust but, in spite of this, tender and, therefore, good for people with sensitive nerves, who tend toward allergic reactions of the skin. Red manuka oil can be applied very well to wounds which do not heal well, eczema, irritated skin and sunburn due to sunshine which is too strong (ozone!). In addition, it is suitable for hay fever and mucous membrane irritations, since the contents work together to stabilize the vegetative nervous system and, thereby, overshooting "allergic reactions".

The strong stabilizing effect on the psyche can be explained by the high content of sesquiterpenes. Through these the oil soothes tense nerves and at the same time strengthens physical and metal resistance.

Mixtures with other ethereal Oils
In combination with tea tree oil and lavender, red manuka has a soothing effect on the irritated scalp even when it tends toward eczema. Together with white manuka, red manuka reduces rheumatism pains, and when cajeput is added an optimal synergetic effect for treating sicknesses of the respiratory pathway is obtained. These ethereal mixtures can be applied directly or used in the aroma lamp.

In place of red manuka, one can use myrrh oil.

Red Manuka Honey

Honey is not only a general, beloved food, but also has many contents such as vitamins, minerals, and trace elements with a high nutritional value and healing properties. It is the only known indestructible food and was used in most of the old cultures not only in foods, but also in medical and cosmetic preparations.

Honey is an ancient, efficient healing agent for almost everything. Because of its properties it was used in countless medicines for treating rickets, scurvy, anemia, rheumatism, migraines, dizziness, constipation, liver, stomach and intestine problems as well as bacterial gastro-enteritis. Its low moisture and high calcium content make it an unsuitable nutrient for the growth of bacteria. It is also used for boils, wounds and burns which threaten to become infected and additionally in infectious diseases, especially of the respiratory pathway.

In our century the "inhibitors" are considered to be responsible for the anti bacterial factors. These are anti bacterial, heat and light sensitive compounds which either inhibit germ reproduction or even kill bacteria. They have been found especially in the dark colored honey varieties, whose main source is not flower nectar but honey dew, which is sucked out of leaves and needles by bees.

The Special Advantages of Red Manuka Honey

Honey has too little water and a too acidic pH value (the human digestive system neutralizes this) for micro-organisms to use. The anti bacterial properties are explained by the glucose-oxidase-enzyme, which leads to the formation of hydrogen peroxide. Red manuka honey, whose anti bacterial activity is approximately 15 – 30% that of phenol, belongs to one of the very rare honey types, where this effect cannot be explained by the hydrogen peroxide factors but through other plant components.

For this reason, red manuka honey can be used therapeutically for all types of infections, (for example, for inhibition of "band worm", cuts, burns, and boils) where it inhibits bacterial reproduction. This has also been observed in wounds where conventional antibiotic and antiseptic remedies showed no effect. *Staphylococcus aures,* for example, which is responsible in part for many cases of wound sepsis in hospitals, and is resistant to most of the antibiotics, can be fought with the anti bacterial effect of honey very effectively without use of peroxide.

Let us not forget that red manuka honey is an extremely strong honey with an intensive aroma. By the way, white manuka is usually there also, since both New Zealand tea trees grow next to one another and their honey is very similar. We use red manuka honey not only to improve the taste of herb teas but also for a softened application of "bitter pills" such as black cumin powder.

White Manuka

White manuka is another "wonder tea tree" from New Zealand. It is very similar to red manuka, but has its own therapeutic focal points.

The Plants

The botanical name is *Leptospermum ericoides,* but designation today is usually under *Kunzea ericoides. Kanuka* is the Maori and German name. It is very similar to red manuka, but is larger (up to 45 feet) and is bushier. It is covered with uncountable white blossoms which grow in bunches and probably give it the name "white manuka". The tree can reach a very old age (more than 150 years) and blooms every year.

Among the native Maoris, the white manuka is particularly valued because of its effect by rheumatism and joint pains, which occur often in warm humid areas with heavy rainfall and corresponding temperature drops.

Contents

The volatile oil is thin, yellow-green and has a very strong smell. 1.6 – 2 tones of leaves yield 1 quart of volatile oil by steam distillation. It is then combined with red manuka to New Zealand "tea tree oil".

The sesquiterpene (cadinene) and sesquiterpene (viridiflorol) are very soothing to the skin and affect messenger components which control the hormonal equilibrium. White Manuka oil has an extremely high content of monoterpenes, which has given it its reputation as an effective anti rheumatism medication.

Special Applications

Even the early settlers used boiled white manuka for the treatment of wounds from cuts and burns as well as for mouth sores by gargling. The leaves were put in hot water and the vapors inhaled for colds and coughs.

Its anti bacterial and fungus effect is weaker than that of tea tree and red manuka. Apart from its decongestive effect by bronchitis and coughs as well as application by all kinds of skin problems (including allergic reactions), white manuka has the mentioned anti rheumatic effect which compares with that of cortisone. By activating the adrenal glands, infection is inhibited and pain reduced.

In addition to its physical effects, white manuka also has a positive effect on spiritual strength and has, especially with red manuka, a psychic stabilizing influence. In aroma therapy it can be combined with lavender, sandal wood and all lemon oils.

As replacement for white manuka one uses pine or incense oil.

From *Die Geheimnisse des Teebaums (The Secrets of the Tea Tree)* we want to end our discourse over the first of the "Three Great Healers" with a citation from Susan Drury:

"The basic message about tea tree oil is that here we have one of the most marvellous healing resources that Nature has to offer..."

—and to extend this Nevill Drury:

"There is no doubt that tea tree oil is a substance which will certainly find its place on the world market for natural healing medications and this demand will increase."

We are convinced that the two Australians at the end of the 80's correctly saw its future.

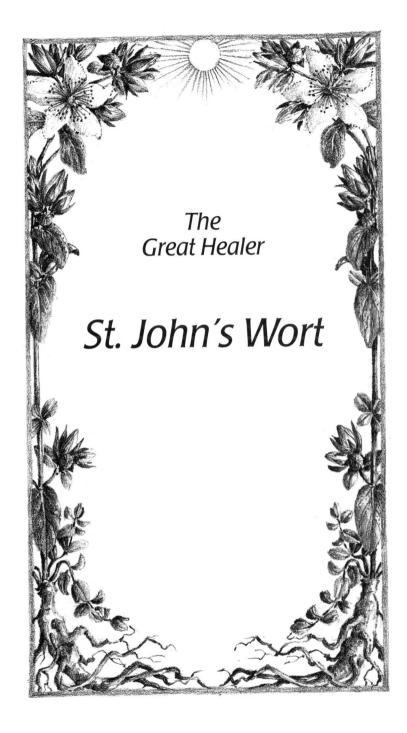

The
Great Healer

St. John's Wort

The very long and lively relationship that binds us with St. John's wort shows no signs of rust. In ancient times, the first day of summer was celebrated with the alchemist's transformation of an oil made from fresh flowers to a ruby red color. The astonishment over this wonder may have contributed to our fidelity throughout the centuries to it. And it was amazing as this herb with its unrelenting inner softness became the number one, anti depressive, plant medication in the course of the last ten years! The many other applications for this many-sided healing plant, which have been recognized by *all* medical directions, have been pushed somewhat into the background. Therefore, we would like to portray the fullness of the great healing applications which are "as important to basic medicine as flour is to bread".

The Plant

St. John's worth belongs to the plant group *Guttiferales* (having oil glands) and the family St. John's wort (*Guttiferae; Hypericaceae*) of the genus *Hypericum* which includes some 380 species. About a third of these have dark secretion containers, which are indicative of the presence of the main active component *hypericin.* The leaves, flowers and other parts of the entire plant family have conspicuous glands in which the volatile oils, resin and balsam are contained.

Our herb, St. John's worth, *Hypericum perforatum,* is a typical, native plant, but by no means limited to our latitudes. It is found throughout North and South America, Europe, the Canary Islands, north Africa, large parts of Asia, China, Australia and New Zealand. The persevering plants are 12 – 30 inches (30 – 72 cm) high, some to 6 feet (2 m), and like company. Light and dry places such as paths, field ridges, forest edges, dry meadows and sunny slopes are preferred. They love light and give it further;

their essence has been described in natural healing as "a warm and dry nature with subtle substance."

St. John's worth has a very straight stem which divides at the top and has a *double* edge—which is very unusual in the plant world. The deep boring, strong roots are similar to a spindle and strongly branched. The leaves are long, oval and smooth-edged. The flowers stand in simple umbela, are sonny, gold yellow, usually in groups of five (seldom with four like clover). They have a weak balsam smell, taste like resin and are slightly bitter, pulling the mouth together.

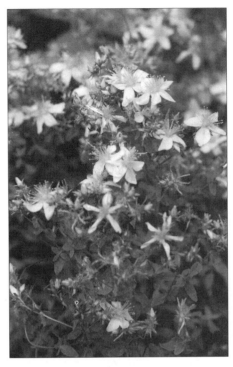

St. John's Wort
(Hypericum perforatum)

They bloom from June to August, particularly in July. In ancient times they were gathered on the longest day when the sun reached its highest point, June 21; with the advent of Christianity this was shifted to St. John's day, June 24. A seed capsule forms from the flowers. The seeds are ripe in August/September; earlier they were gathered for healing purposes on August 15, the day that Mary ascended into heaven.

When one observes the plant against the light, the leaves look as though they were perforated; which explains the Latein name *Hypericum "perforatum"*. But these so called holes are glands which contain the volatile oil. Even the finely pointed, lanceolate sepals and the actual petals of the blossoms have black tips; the petals dark violet stripes. When the fresh flowers are squeezed between the fingers, a blood red juice emerges. Its color comes from the main active component of St. John's wort, hypericin, which is the base of the thousand year long fascination with this worthy plant and its healing properties.

Hypericum perforatum

The German name "Johanniskraut" and the English name St. John's wort come from Christian legends while the Latin name *perforatum* was first documented in a list of drugs used by the famous medical teaching staff from Salerno. The name *hypericum* was used by the ancient Romans. In Greek it is *perikón* or *hypereikon*. Later authors neglected to explain the name or invented reasons for it. From *hypo* = "over" and *eikon* = "picture" arose a number of interpretations, for example:
* botanical: the light secretion containers in the leaves of the plant is a picture (which is beyond the imagination)
* medical: the plant has healing powers beyond every picture (or every idea)
* spiritual-religious: the plant transfers experiences which go beyond every picture or conception. These pictures deal with the subconscious or with the world of evil spirits and inner demons, which the herb should fight according to old superstitions.

We personally tend toward the interpretation that the *Hypericum* species of the plant has been hung *above the pictures* of gods to repel bad spirits since ancient times. That this is apparently true even today, is shown in the experience of a friend, whose favorite plant is St John's wort:

Our forefathers used St. John's wort against "bad spirits." I convinced myself of the effect of this sunny herb myself. One day, our daughter who was 1 1/2 years old at that time, starred with a fearful face into an apparent emptiness. With horror I saw that an over dimensional being with cold boring glance was between us. The atmosphere was very unpleasant. Even friends who visited us found this ghastly. After this being bothered us every day and tortured our daughter, whose cries of fear we heard again and again nights, we attempted to alter her mood with St. John's wort in the following manner:

St. John's wort was mixed with sage in the ratio of 2:1 and the house filled with the vapors. We hung a large bouquet of St. John's wort in almost every room. The results were singular: we had peace from this figure, whose mere presence flooded us with misgivings! Another comment: the effect does not disappear with the process of drying. Even in Winter, one can drive the "bad spirits" away with the beautiful dry bouquets or wreaths from St. John's wort..

Hypericum Species—a large number of Relatives

In Europe, there are about a dozen main species which occur (in the world there are several hundred). In addition to the common St. John's wort *Hypericum perforatum* which is called *Tüpfel-Johanniskraut* "dotted St. John's wort", there is the spotted St. John's wort (*hypericum maculatum),* which is also named *Hypericum quadrangulum* after its four-sided stem, the winged version *H. tetrapterum* and the low lying *H. humifusum,* the haired *H. hirsutum,* or bearded *H. barbatum,* the beautiful *H. pulchrum,* the delicate *H. elegans,* the swamp *H. elodes,* and mountain *H. montanum* Even by the common St. John's wort there is a small and large leafed type (*H. perf. sp angusti-folium + latifolium*) as well as the subdivision *Hypericum veronese*.

In the United States, in addition to common St. John's wort, there are a number of other species with character-istics corresponding to those in Europe. These include spotted St. John's wort with leaves and flowers conspicu-ously dotted with black (H. punctatum), coppery St. John's wort with a 4-angled stem (H. denticulatum), Canadian St. John's wort with narrow leaves and which is up to 20 inches high (H. canadense), Arons's beard or the Rose of Sharon (H. calycinum), and the pale St. John's wort up to 20 inch-es and found in marshes (H. ellipticum). Among the more common species are two shrubby St. John's worts, one with woody, 2-edged twigs (H. spathulatum) and one with narrower leaves and 5 styles (H. Kalmianum), a golden St. John's wort with smaller deep yellow flowers (H. patulum), the dwarf St. John's wort with oval leaves and up to 3 feet heigh (H. mutilum) and the great St. John's wort with 2 inch leaves and flowers reaching heights of up to 6 feet (H. py-ramidatum).

It can easily happen that the St John's wort which one gathers oneself and puts in a herb tea or oil does not turn red when put in the sun. One is very disappointed. For-tunately there are more criteria by which the herbs can be differentiated, so that with time one can find the *real* St. John's wort:

❀ It generally prefers a dry place.

❀ When one holds the plant against the light, the leaves appear to be perforated because of the oil glands.

❀ The flowers have black dots and dark violet stripes. When pressed, a juice is released which colors the fin-gers crimson red.

❀ The most clear characteristic is the double edged stem since even if the other characteristics are similar, the stem by its relatives is either round or four sided.

The Medicine of cleaver Men and Women

A Legendary Plant with many Names

There are almost more common names for St. John's wort in Germany than in botany. Particular significance is attached to St. John's day, the day when John the Baptist was born (incidentally, it is exactly half a year before Christmas, the day on which Christ was born). This date is three days after the solstice, the day on which the sun reaches it's highest point in the sky, June 21. These coincidences, not only identify St. John's wort as a plant which captures the full energy of the sun, but also is in full bloom on St. John's Day when it is traditionally picked (it plays an important role in the customs of this day). The relationship between the red plant juice and the blood that St John the Baptist lost when he was beheaded is drawn so that names such as *Johannisblut* "John's blood" and *Johannisschweiß* "John's sweat" have been derived. The blood motive is also a rich source for names such as *Blutkraut* "blood herb", *Mannsblutkraut* "man's blood herb", *Elfenblutkraut* or *Alfblut* "elf blood herb", as well as *Christusblut* "Christ's blood".

Its use as a wound healing medication derived from the blood red juice has also inspired many names such as balm-of-warrior, *Wundkraut* "wound herb", or *Unseres Herrgotts Wundenkraut* "Our Lord's wound herb", and the simplified versions *Herrgottskraut* "Lord's herb" or Grace of God.

The botanical characteristics of the plant are also preserved in names such as *Hartheu* "hard hay", or more precisely *Tüpfel-Hartheu* "dotted hard hay", which refers to the hard stem of the plant. Naturally the perforations have left their traces as in *Durchbohrten Johanniskraut* "pierced St John's wort", *Löcherlkraut* "hole herb" or the French

Mille pertuis and the Italian *mille bucchi* "thousand hole herb". The name *fuga daemonum* "devil's curse" comes from the tale that the devil was so angry about the wonderful power of the herb that he punched a thousand needle holes through it in the hope of killing it; but he only succeeded in strengthening the legendary healing effect thereby.

Many customs that we would today relegate to the edges of magic and "superstition" such as protection from pistol bullets, wounds, storms, lightning as well as its use in prophesies about love and the future, probably have their roots here. Since Paracelsus, the demons have been moved within and equated with "fantasising" or psychic

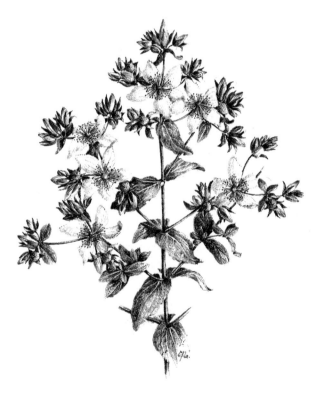

Drawing of St. John's wort

disturbances from melancholy to obsession. As we know, St John's wort is *the* natural healing medication for treating depression.

A number of other names from common botany acknowledge the medical healing effect such as *Nabelkraut* "belly button herb" or *Liefwehbloom* "pain away flower" as a result of the effects in the area of the stomach and the solar plexus; *Frauenkraut* "woman's herb" or *Liebfrauen-Bettstroh* "Virgin Mary's bed straw" based on the role that it plays by women's suffering (the names *Mannskraft* "man's power" and *Liebeskraut* "love herb") have also been handed down; *Waldhopfenkraut* "forest hop herb" or *Fieldhopfenkraut* "field hop herb" as a result of its soothing sleep etc. Another set of names mirrors its broad application spectrum and honor such as *Wildgartheil* "wild garden healing" or *Allheil* "all healing"; In English tutsan or touch-and-heal; In French *Toute Sainte* (all holy). With this attribute we close our small detour.

Ancient Healing Herb with astonishing Advantages

A healing plant with so many descriptive names, will never be neglected like a wall-flower. St John's herb was called "Cheiron's root" and appears as *hypericum* or *hypereikon* by all of the Greek and roman authors in the area of natural history and medicine such as Hippocrates, Pliny and Dioscorides. Several, at least four, species were distinguished on the basis of their botanical characteristics but not differentiated with respect to their healing effects. According to the old writings, the main active substance was the red coloring hypericin, which was known at that time as *androsaimon* (man's blood), indicative of its use for wounds. At the same time it stopped bleeding, killed germs, reduced pain, hindered infection and aided healing. Burns, contusions, dirty sores and all badly healed wounds were treated at that time with the blood red St John's wort oil; it was also recommended for massage by sciatic and rheumatic pains. Oil, tea and various tinctures were used against worms, digestive disturbances, for strengthening the heart and liver, removing gall and cleaning the kidneys, by lung sicknesses and congestion, and as a many-sided help for women. As a result of its many applications, Albertus Magnus and after him Conrad von Megenberg praised it as a "king's crown".

St. John's wort was the favorite plant of Paracelsus, who raised it to prominence because of its mental effects which he called "Phantasmata". Apart from *perforata* he named only corals as a medication against sicknesses whereby "a person was ruled by another spirit." Melancholy was seen as an "inner demon", which we refer to as a depression today. This explanation for mood sicknesses is not at all unusual as our expression "be something better" shows. Customarily in the Orient, evil spirits or demons are considered responsible for physical sicknesses. The famous Sinologist Richard Wilhelm (I Ging) even called the fear of bacteria a "modern form of belief in sprits (interestingly enough, St. John's wort has not only an anti depressive effect but also an anti bacterial effect).

In his *Pflantengeheimnissen* "Plant Secrets", Willy Schroedter found according to the homeopathic principle for similarities:

> *In St. John's wort is a good spirit.*
> *The "St. John spirit" helps against destructive*
>   *spirits (bacteria).*
> *One sprit fights another spirit.*

St. John's wort takes on a new Profile

When we return to the facts, it becomes evident that St John's wort appeared in all the great plant encyclopaedias of the 16th to 18th century from Hieronymus Bock to *Tabernaemontanus,* as a cure for internal and external wounds. The many names and prescriptions show that it was well known, loved and had many applications. At the beginning of the 19th century it was referred to in a medical practice book as "the very famous wound medicine." We can conclude that as a result of the victories of technical and medical progress, even such a "king's crown" was neglected for a while. From the French Revolution to the Industrial Revolution, it was used less and less. St. John's wort was even called a "placebo," after Shikonine was substituted for it on the market.

Research with the real red active substance hypericin has continued. Despite the centuries of use, biochemistry, pharmacology and medicine are attempting to establish if, why and how it works. The more substances studied, whose scientific effectiveness is established, the more it has regained its favor, so that in the middle of our century it was rediscovered as a nerve medication as well as an emergency medication by burns. In the last decade it has had a Renaissance.

Today a number of pharmacological firms manufacture medicines containing St. John's wort or hypericin, some in combination with other medications. It is available dried for making tea, in pulverized form or as a liquid, in capsules, as pills, as a solution for injection and as fresh plant, pressed juice. St John's wort oil can be obtained either as a liquid or as a salve for external application as well as oil capsules for internal use. *Herba hyperici* is in the valid "Deutsches Arzneibuch" (German medicine book, DAB 9) and "Deutscher Arzneimittel-Codex" (German medicine code, DAC 1986/1995) with a special commentary on plant medications by Commission E, which is responsible for standard approval. The astonishing, thereby, is not the large demand and spread of this wound and soul balsam but the fact that natural healing and school medicine, plant and psycho therapists, nervous old women and young herb witches, seldom are in such agreement as in this case. Doesn't this make you curious about the contents of the plant which is capable of such a wonder?

Active Ingredients and Contents of St. John's wort

The old healing knowledge based on experience and common practice rests on the principle *"Who (or what) heals is right"*. The question of whether a healing plant is a medicine or a poison, was answered by Paracelsus, as being dependent on the correct dosage.

Nature, the great teacher, provides no isolated "single drugs" but mixtures, which are referred to in our age as "complex medications". Today one demands from plant medications not only the same requirements for the "proof of quality, effectiveness and harmlessness" as for chemically synthesized medications, but one also attempts to determine the individual active component(s). This isn't easy and one is often unsatisfied with the results, since it is known that the whole is more than the sum of its parts. A complex medication is more than just a complex effect: the effect is magnified by the "synergetic effect" of many-sided and different contents.

In order to obtain scientific proof of its effectiveness, the mixture from the plant extract is separated into its individual components by being run through a separation column. In succeeding experiments it is determined which of the individual components has effects resembling most closely that of the mixture.

It is unbelievable: for many healing plants, the active components which are responsible for the effects are not yet or not completely known. In such cases, quality control is based on the distinguishing components, the so-called "guiding substances".

Precisely this paradoxical case has happened with St. John's wort: the anti depressive effect has been conclusively established, but the components responsible for it still aren't known. Up until recently it had been believed that hypericin, which is the "guiding substance" in the available preparations, was responsible for these effects.

Although we suspect that the effectiveness of St. John's wort as an anti depressive depends on the synergetic effects of a number of components, we will describe hypericin which may be the most important component of St. John's wort.

Hypericin: Legend and Reality

The dark red juice from the transparent oil glands and the fresh blossoms is responsible for legends about the "wonder plant". The mysterious red dye in St. John's wort, which was once called "hypericum red", was first called hypericin in 1911, although it was not conclusively isolated until 1939. Hypericin is dissolved in the cell juice and is found not only in the secretion containers of the blossoms, but after the seeds are ripe in all parts of the plant except the roots and fruit.

Hypericin is a dianthrone and is almost always found in St. John's wort together with related compounds, particularly pseudohypericin. Plants have about 0.1 – 0.3% hypericin. The ratio of hypericin to related compounds in the plant and the extracts is about 6/4.

Hypercin is a light sensitive substance, which has an effect on the messenger substances in the brain. It causes the production of melatonin in the pineal gland which counteracts the inner winter depression resulting from less light as well as general depressive moods. Hypericin is also known as mycoporphyrin and behaves similarly to the body's porphyrins, for example hematoporphyrin, which is formed in the body as a decomposition product of hemoglobin.

People who react oversensitively to light should be careful when using St. John's wort, although this effect of hypericin occurs only in sunlight. In the presence of light and oxygen, photo-oxidation of cell components can result from this photo-dynamic effect; in extreme cases this can lead to hemolysis (break down) of the red blood cells. Light skinned sheep, cows and horses have been found to suffer from sunburn-like swelling, infections, boils and hair loss after eating quantities of St. John's wort. The symptoms are known as *hypericismus*. However, usually photo toxic or allergic symptoms are only observed in light skinned humans after very intensive sun exposure and/or a large overdose.

The Antibiotic Hyperforin

In addition, St. John's wort contains 2 – 4% phloroglucin derivatives, among them the anti bacterial hyperforin which is comparatively concentrated in the fresh blossoms, buds, and seed capsules, and contributes to the antibiotic effectiveness as a wound healing medication. Hyperforin is chemically similar to the bitter components of hops, humulon and lupulon and is probably involved in the soothing effect of the herb.

Flavones and Bioflavonoids

Flavones and bioflavonoids are the next active components in St. John's wort, accounting for about 2 – 4%. *Quercetin (glucoside)*, which is one of the most widespread flavones in the plant kingdom is the dominant component. It is thought to have an inhibitory effect on the enzyme monoaminoxydase (MAO), which is important for brain metabolism and hormone synthesis. The flavonoid *camperol* and the flavonoid-glycoside *hyperosid* (which was often confused earlier with the yellow dye "hyperin" as well as other flavone compounds) are involved in the broad application spectrum of the complex medication.

The flavonoids are basic components of many natural yellow plant dyes. They are usually bound chemically on a bitter glycoside, but their effect has not yet been fully explained. Recent research indicates that they have a large impact on the immune system and the body's protection mechanisms. They fight certain bacteria and viruses, which is why they are used for infections. Many of them inhibit infection and serve as anti oxidants against "free radicals." Flavonoids even have the ability to repair capillaries and cell membranes (without side effects) so that they hinder the spread of many sicknesses. One calls this the reduction-oxidation system.

Further Contents

St. John's wort contains between 4 and more than 16 % tannins, which are concentrated most strongly in the flowers. These are primarily built from catechin elements. These are the same building blocks which are found in *Catechu* and *Cola* species which are found in green tea. It is possible that they even have an effect on digestion. Apart from hypericin, hyperosid and natural chlorophyll, the presence of the flower dye cyanidin has been established. *Procyanidine,* which is also found in hawthorn and is known for its ability to strengthen the heart—is supported by the flavonoids and tannins. Finally a number of diverse *plant acids* are found in St. John's wort, among them ascorbic acid (vitamin C).

The Volatile Oil

Both the light and dark secretion containers in the leaves of St. John's wort have a clear, viscose secretion, primarily a mixture of volatile oil and resin. They give St. John's wort the apparently perforated structure. The amount of volatile oil is extremely small (0.1 – 0.3%); so that it cannot be distilled by the usual procedures but must be distilled by a tedious special procedure. For this reason volatile St. John's wort is a very expensive rarity. For the same reason, it is seldom mentioned in aroma therapy literature, although it contains extremely effective active components, which strengthen as well as round off the complex effect of St. John's wort.

The light yellow to light green volatile oil has a pleasant herb smell with a light fir tree note. Almost 30 chemical compounds could be established to date, mainly sesquiterpenes, aromatic aldehydes and monoterpene alcohols, among them alpha and beta pinene, limonene, humulene, caryophyllene, alpha-terpineol, geraniol, etc. The ethereal oil has special cramp dissolving and blood coagulating, infection inhibiting, and wound healing properties, which are strengthened by the combined effect with the dye components. In addition it has an effect on the mucous membrane and the solar plexus. This very special mixture is responsible for the favorable influence of post traumatic processes and shock and has given St. John's wort the name of "arnica of the nerves".

Pure ethereal St. John's wort oil should be used internally and externally only in very dilute form. It is also ideal in an aroma lamp. Attention: always make an allergy test first!

St. John's Wort—the secret of its Effect

Enough of the isolated substances, now to the complex medication St. John's wort. The synergetic composition of all known and unknown components gives St. John's wort its extraordinary effect. It works on the interaction of the nervous system and hormone secretion, circulation and digestion and is also above all the medication when "the soul lies broken on the ground"—as the herb pastor Weidinger picturesquely expressed it. The *sum* of the contents stimulates the glands of the digestion organs and the gall-bladder, works normalizing on the inner hormone gland system and stimulates the circulation. St. John's wort is *the* nerve-soul rebuilding medication. It also has a light soothing effect on body and soul as a result of the very special mixture of relaxing and activating effects but it does not make anything apathetic.

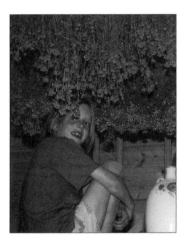

A good St. John's wort harvest is a balsam for body and soul

What Properties does St. John's Wort have?

Here are the great positive points for St. John's wort—in combination with its main applications:
* antibacterial and anti viral (wound treatment, colds)
* anthelmintic (destroying or expelling intestinal worms)
* internal and external infection inhibiting (local antiphogistic, wound treatment, skin care)
* pain reducing (wound treatment; nerve pains and neuralgia)

- ❀ reducing bleeding (wound treatment)
- ❀ protecting capillaries (wound treatment, skin care)
- ❀ softens irritations (stomach; nervous system)
- ❀ stimulates secretion (stomach, intestine, liver, gall-bladder, glands and hormones)
- ❀ stimulates menstruation (regulative effect)
- ❀ relieves cramps (stomach-intestine, bladder, colics)
- ❀ induces urine (kidneys, bladder, colics, stone formation)
- ❀ dissolves slime (colds, lungs/bronchi, asthma)
- ❀ soothing and relaxing (nerves, head and heart; neuralgia and nerve pain).

As Antidepressant in Vogue

For a long time St. John's wort was only known as a red oil for external use in the treatment of wounds. Its effect as a nerve medication and antidepressant when applied internally has only recently been rediscovered. For this reason, this aspect forms the focal point of our interest.

The Effect on Brain Metabolism and the Nervous System

It is scientifically proven that depressed people have a disturbed biochemical equilibrium which prevents the brain from operating optimally. This can lead to mental, spiritual and emotional disturbances as well as physical disturbances which fall under the heading of "depression".

The human brain is the finest and most complex communication center that we know. A hundred thousand million brain cells transmit billions of messages every second. These biochemical transmission substances are known as messenger components or *neuro transmitters*. When they are available in the required quantity, the brain functions harmoniously and can establish the necessary equilibrium despite high demands. When certain neurotransmitters are lacking, one can be thrown out of his central position. On one hand this can cause a feeling of depression let down, on the other hand it can lead to an increase of certain substances, stress symptoms or manic states of arousal.

Alan Watts, the famous, new-age philosopher, said that the brain causes all of this without our thinking about it at all. But although the brain functions without our consciousness, we can do something about the brain metabolism to re-establish the biochemical equilibrium. This is the basis for the synthetic and plant anti depressive medications. St. John's wort is one of the softest medications for this. According to the latest research, it works at the following circuits in the brain:

❀ St. John's wort affects the messenger compound *dopamine,* which regulates the hormone adrenaline and neurotranmitter noradrenaline. It inhibits nerve signals so that the psychic equilibrium is re-established. St. John's wort stabilizes dopamine so that the so-called "stress hormone" noradrenaline is not released. As a result of the effect on the brain centers for processing, irritations are shielded. The irritating flood is stopped so that the mental/-spiritual and physical thresholds are increased.

❀ Another basis is the effect on the pineal gland at the base of the brain, which among other things, regulates the release of the hormone *melatonin.* When there is not enough light, for example in winter, too much melatonin may be released during the day so that the disturbed rhythm leads to sleepiness, irritability and depressive symptoms. This is the case in the typical "winter depression."

❀ Another switch in the brain which is influenced by St. John's wort is "MAO" the enzyme monoaminoxydase. St. John's wort inhibits the enzyme MAO, which itself inhibits the activity of the neurotransmitter *serotonin* in the brain. This is an activity which should be as free and uninhibited as possible because: serotonin is a type of "happy hormone" releasing substances which reduce pain and allow one to fall asleep.

To put it simply, St. John's wort provides a shield against the irritation flood and reduces excitability as well as strengthening the nerves, brightening the mood, increasing the initiative almost to ecstasy on one hand but on the other causing a psychic stability so that one can better cope with the stress situation, the mental demands, the pressure for accomplishment, large burdens and fears. St. John's wort is not only a plant "tranquilizer" but also dissolves depressive symptoms when taken for an extended period.

The Mental-Spiritual Signature

St. John's wort is a medication for internal and external wounds. Its mental-spiritual effect reaches a central significance. It has captured the full power of the sun at its highest position in the year. This makes it a *light plant*. With all its leaves, it adsorbs the light energy and stores it in the compounds contained in the secretion containers and oil glands. It grows straight and strong while being firmly anchored in the ground.

From this plant signature, one can conclude that it is very compatible for those who long for the inner light but easily give up and worry because they lack the bright, sunny confidence and strength to overcome their problems. This point of view is that of the allopathic effect. Homeopathically seen, these people constantly stand in the spotlight so that their nerves are torn and they become stressed and sometimes "loose their nerves." Those whose continuous activity leads to nervous exhaustion and sleep disturbances also belong to this group. In their case, this can lead to a reduced tension between the nerves and muscle or lead to cramps. St John's wort with its many-sided application possibilities can give all these types inner relaxation and real strength—not just an external support.

St. John's Wort in Homeopathy

St. John's wort is considered to be "the arnica of the nerves" in homeopathy and is used primarily for the peripheral and central nervous systems.

Mother liquid (and D1):
- ❀ externally for support of wound treatment especially after injury of the nerve endings; also for open wounds and haemorrhoids
- ❀ by nerve infections, nerve damage by trauma and traumatic neuroses
- ❀ is supported by internal consumption of low to middle potencies.

middle potency 3 (C3 or D6):
- ❀ internally to soothe the nerves, as a light sleep inducer or against sleepiness and mild anti depressive agent; against fears, uncertainty and stage fright
- ❀ anemic conditions with headaches at the top of the head and circulation disturbances
- ❀ with numb feelings after nerve injury, post traumatic processes, by brain and spinal cord shock
- ❀ for bladder cramps, hemorrhoid bleeding, vagina infections and infections of the uterus membrane
- ❀ congestion, for example in the brain, heart, and lungs
- ❀ asthma attacks
- ❀ dizziness or equilibrium disturbances

higher potencies:
- ❀ seldom, only by tedious chronic disturbances with clear-cut key symptoms.

Most Recent Research

Since St. John's wort has moved to a point of central interest and its main anti depressive active components are being studied, a number of studies and research experiments have opened the following new application possibilities:

- ❀ inhibition of the growth of retroviren such as HIV virus (AIDS) and FV virus (leukaemia)
- ❀ inhibition of certain forms of tumor growth (for example, brain tumors) by cell regulation (redox)
- ❀ inhibition of the hepatitis C virus (HCV)
- ❀ sterilization of donor blood by blood transfusions as well as
- ❀ ulcers, skin diseases and rheumatic arthritis.

Recommended Applications

As opposed to psycho drugs and anti depressives, which require a prescription, side effects very seldom occur with St. John's wort; when they do, they disappear immediately after the medication is discontinued. In very few cases—and then usually by an over dose—stomach-intestine reactions or allergic symptoms can occur. One of these is a skin infection resembling sunburn after exposure to very strong sun radiation (caution: solarium!) of light skinned persons with an over sensitivity to light. It is precisely the photosensitivity effect on the skin which influences the better use of light and, thereby, the serotonin and melatonin metabolism. The already mentioned *hypericismus* by slight skinned animals does not occur in humans—not even when one is injected with hypericum. Naturally after rubbing St. John's wort oil into the skin, one shouldn't lie in the sun for a while!

- ❀ St. John's wort is compatible with all other medications (with the possible exception of MAO inhibitors).
- ❀ In order to brighten the mood, it is necessary to take the herb for at least 4 – 6 weeks up to 2 – 3 months.
- ❀ To increase the effect, injections of hyperforat are recommended at the beginning.

Correct Dosage is Important

❀ *Capsules or solution*
Up to 30 drops or 2 capsules 3 times a day; after 14 days, 20 drops or 1 capsule twice a day
❀ *Freshly pressed plant juice*
1 – 2 tablespoons (eventually diluted) 3 times a day; after 14 days 1 tablespoon (eventually diluted) mornings and evenings
❀ *St. John's wort oil (for internal use)*
1 tablespoon eventually diluted 2 – 3 times a day
❀ *St. John's wort as tea*
about 3 cups per day; in mixtures almost unlimited

Making your own St. John's Wort Oil

Many of our friends and acquaintances and, of course, we ourselves, make fresh St. John's wort oil every year with great enthusiasm. According to old reports, the best harvesting times are naturally St. John's day (June 24) before the dew or at 12 midday; also a few days before or after the next full moon as well as days that it blooms on which the moon is in an astrological air sign. In any case, one must be certain that the plant (preferably in undisturbed nature) is completely dry when it is

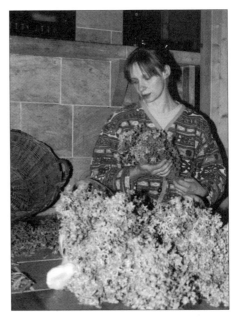

St. John's wort is processed while it is still fresh right after it is gathered.

75

gathered (so that the oil doesn't develop mold later). To be certain that the oil turns ruby red in the sun, one should read page 57 about how one can be certain that one has the real *Hypericum perforatum.* The blossoms and buds are pulled from very fresh plants and put into a wide mouthed, white glass container and fully covered with your favorite oil pressed at ambient temperature. You should make enough for one year. There are several variations of how to proceed:

❀ The glass container is covered with a paper or gauze so that the air can get in and placed in the sun. After about 4 – 6 weeks the oil turns ruby red.

❀ First the glass container is placed open in a warm place to ferment and stirred daily. Then close the container and place in the sun (as before).

❀ In order to increase the active ingredients, after about 14 days when the oil begins to turn red, press the flowers and replace with freshly gathered flowers. This can be repeated several times to increase the active contents.

❀ after a few weeks when the oil is an intensive red color, filter through a cloth and press the flowers with your hands. Now carefully pour the oil out, separating it from the water layer.

❀ pour into small (30 – 50 ml) bottles which are not transparent to light and store in the dark.

Usually olive oil pressed at ambient temperature is used for making St. John's wort *wound oil.* In order to make it longer lasting it is mixed with a good thistle oil. Sunflower oil is not to be recommended because it easily becomes rancid. For certain uses, smaller amounts can be made with the type of oil selected for a stronger "synergetic effect". Here are a few examples:

❀ *linseed oil* special for burns

❀ *wheat germ oil* for skin care

❀ *pumpkin seed oil* for bladder problems and bed wetting

❀ *black cumin seed oil* for stomach problems

- ❀ *sesame oil* as concentrated nerve supplement
- ❀ *hemp oil* for muscle and joint pains as well as by gall bladder problems

and certainly there are many other suitable combinations—according to experience and dependent on the effects that one wants to reach.

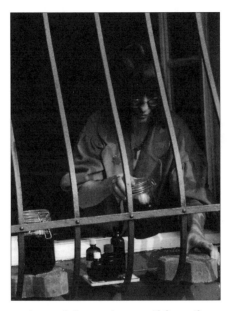

A special experience: oil from the yellow blossoms turns ruby red.

THE BEST APPLICATIONS FOR ST. JOHN'S WORT

Directions for use and prescriptions can be found in the appendix "Uses from A – Z"

External Applications

St. John's wort relates very closely with the skin—not just because the skin is "the mirror of the soul" but because the light sensitive effect enfolds over it. Many of its properties are excellent for the treatment of wounds, skin problems, and skin care, because it is antibacterial, stills blood, reduces pain, inhibits infections, is astringent, protects and regenerates tissue. Especially St. John's wort oils as well as tinctures, salves and extracts in skin care medications are used for external use and then always effectively supported internally when the nervous system is involved.

Wounds

Especially in the form of oil, St. John's wort is highly antibacterial, as can be shown at high dilutions with *staphylococcus aureas*. Its antiseptic properties almost always prevent the formation of pus. It pulls together and supports regeneration of the injured skin tissue. Usually it heals completely without leaving a scar.

We aren't the only ones who have positive experiences with
* burns
* blows, bites and cuts
* bleeding wounds
* effusion of blood
* bruises and contusions

Without having to wash the—even dirty—wounds, a thick (gauze bandage) compression soaked in St. John's wort oil is laid over it. Important: the wound must always be kept wet and oily so that it doesn't dry out. For this reason the compression should be changed several times a day. Further disinfection is reached when, *St. John's wort tincture* made with ethanol is used.

Despite its long history, its special effectiveness with burns has never been forgotten. For this application, it is best to use St. John's wort oil made with linseed oil, which is in itself effective by burns and increases the synergetic effect many times. By burns it is especially important to apply the oil as quickly as possible since this increases the chance that no scars remain. The detailed report of our friend gives further details:

St. John's wort, a medication loved by the entire family, appears to help especially by burns. At the age of six years, our son was in intensive care with third degree burns. Every day he was given a special bath which dissolved the bandages and various layers of skin. As far as possible, I dropped St. John's wort oil on the skin areas which weren't bandaged every evening. The results astonished the doctors: the open areas healed much quicker and without forming scars. For us, this was reason enough to spare the poor child the extremely painful baths and to treat him with St. John's wort oil at home. Five years have passed since then and one can't see any evidence of the burns.

St. John's wort is very effective in conbination when used together or alternating with arnica and marigolds as salves or homeopathic mother solutions. Persistent sores, *ulcus cruris,* and wounds which are healing badly with changes in the tissue are receptive to this treatment.

Through the connection between the brain and the nerves, St. John's wort exerts a special effectiveness by all peripheral nerve damage. Post traumatic and post operative pains (amputation stump pains, even after puncturing the spine or extracting teeth). All injuries to areas rich in sensory nerves such as the finger tips, the toes, the base of the spinal column react favorably to this "arnica of the nerves". The pain recedes quickly, the nerves regenerate and let "the light shine through" again. To name a few examples:

- ❀ pierce, cut, or tear wounds caused by nails or splinters in the feet
- ❀ thorns or splinters under the nails
- ❀ pressing or hammering pains in the fingers, toes or under the nails
- ❀ pus accumulation in finger or hand infections
- ❀ sliped disk
- ❀ coccyx contusion (base of the spinal column)
- ❀ nerve pains
- ❀ nerve infections
- ❀ neuralgia (pain along the face nerve trigeminus and migraines; spinal cord/disk)
- ❀ lumbago
- ❀ paralysis and numb feeling

In all these cases treatment can be supported by internally taking St. John's wort. From our own experience we can especially recommend the homeopathic middle potencies 3 (C3 or D6).

In addition it can be used for massage and rubbing in by

- ❀ general weakness of the limbs
- ❀ back aches
- ❀ sprains and dislocations
- ❀ muscle and joint pains
- ❀ rheumatic pains

Skin Care

As a result of the infection inhibiting and astringent properties as well as the ability to regenerate and protect skin tissue, St. John's oil is the ideal balsam for healthy and problematic skin. At the top of the list are the alcoholic solutions or extracts in salves as well as components of skin care agents.

Instructions for your own Preparations

In the preparation of St. John's oil, a particularly skin-compatible oil should be chosen. We have always had good results with wheat germ or almond oil.

One can also easily make a St. John's wort tincture: One lets fresh flowers soak for 10 – 14 days in alcohol. Press them out, strain and store closed tightly. A 40 – 50% alcohol is sufficient; when using a higher percent alcohol (which is necessary for the extraction of certain substances), the tincture should be diluted with distilled water afterwards.

St. John's wort is to be recommended by the following skin problems (please determine if the oil or alcohol preparation is better yourself):
* ❀ itching rash, which becomes worse when cold, wet or touched
* ❀ erythemata (infected redness of the skin caused by hyperamie)
* ❀ psoriasis
* ❀ Herpes (blister rash), Herpes zoster
* ❀ sores and boils
* ❀ acne and seborrhoea

All infections on areas exposed to light , even allergic reactions, profit from the oil. Sunburn has interesting indications:

St. John's wort can itself cause sunburn-similar infections as a result of its photo sensitive properties. Light sensitive, particularly light skinned persons should avoid a high dosage of strong sunlight in summer and not rub in the red oil and lie in the sun. In spite of this: by sunburn the homeopathic principle *"Like heals like"* can be applied because St. John's wort oil is extremely soothing and healing and supports the formation of protective skin pigments.

One could write an entire chapter, if not a book about the components of skin care medications and cosmetics. In this connection, it is interesting that St. John's wort is used as a spagyric component of plant extracts. For blemishes, a tendency toward dandruff flakes or small tears and cracks, raw and especially sensitive skin received through the combination of active substances in St. John's wort a deep rest, which is also a "balsam for the soul".

Recipe for face water for mild skin cleaning
(very good for cleaning especially sensitive skin)

St. John's wort, witch hazel (Hammelis virginia) and wheat germ are mixed in equal portions and put in a wide necked glass container. Add 40% – 90% ethanol in a ratio of 1:4 plants/ethanol. Let it remain at room temperature on the window sill for 14 days. It must be shaken or stirred once each day. Strain (press the solid mass) and dilute to 20% with distilled water.

Internal Application

St. John's wort has an extremely broad spectrum of application as a result of the connection between the nerves and the hormone system, the circulatory and digestive systems. Equally many-sided are the ways of taking it: as tea, juice, tincture, oil, capsules and drops as well as injections. Because of the many possibilities, we present only a summary here. In any case, the appendix "Applications from A – Z" is very inspiring.

Digestion and Excretion

St. John's wort regulates the acidy in the stomach and prevents fermentation. In addition it stimulates digestion, gall bladder function and induces excretion, so that it can be used by the following symptoms:

❀ stomach and intestine discomfort, even if they result from nervousness
❀ stomach-intestine infection, diarrhoea, flatulence (accumulation of gas), and heartburn
❀ stomach catarrh (infection of the stomach mucous membrane, ulcers)
❀ stimulation of digestion (by loss of appetite)
❀ Stimulation of the liver and gall bladder
❀ gall bladder colic
❀ jaundice
❀ dropsy (excessive accumulation of fluid)
❀ kidney and bladder stones, colics
❀ loss of tension of the bladder muscles
❀ bladder cramps and enuresis (incontinence)

Heart and Circulation

St. John's wort balances heart activity (through its effect on the nervous system), increases the blood flow through

the heart muscle and prevents blockage by overfilling. Therefore, it is recommended to take it for
- ❀ heart problems caused by nervousness—heart neurosa
- ❀ disturbed blood circulation
- ❀ congestion in various organs
- ❀ anemia (stimulation of blood formation)
- ❀ weather dependant aches
- ❀ also by asthma and difficulty breathing

Hormone System

Through its effect on brain metabolism and the inner secretory glands, St. John's wort has a far reaching, regulatory influence on hormone balance. It can be applied to many complaints related to them, among them:
- ❀ decreased hormone function—weak menstruation (anemic young women)
- ❀ cramping menstrual pains
- ❀ vagina and uterus infections
- ❀ headaches and migraines caused by hormones
- ❀ menopause (bleeding and depression)

Don't loose your Nerves ...

We wanted to hold the suspense and have withheld the "cream" of the applications till last. St. John's wort is doubtless a psychic healing plant of great effectiveness, not a tranquilizer which relaxes, but one which reaches deep into the soul, brightens the mood and has a clear stabilizing effect.

We shouldn't forget that it is a relatively gentle "anti depressive" whose effects are neither as quick nor as intense and clear as those of synthetic psycho drugs and anti depressives. For this reason, St. John's wort is not the right medication for heavy, depressions which result from inner malfunctions, but by light to middle reactive and neurotic forms. It is also necessary to take it for an extended time span.

Depressions often go unrecognized and are, therefore, one of the most underestimated and untreated illnesses. Even when obvious "negative" indications are lacking, many people feel depressed by the lack of "positive" impulses. The most basic depressive symptom is medically termed *Anhedonie* and manifests itself through apathy, lack of enjoyment of life and more or less permanent dissatisfaction.

This feeling is found in almost all Woody Allen films, and especially in the characters he portrays himself. An example is found in the dialogue to his film *Annie Hall,* who with respect to her symptoms could have been called *Annie Hedonia:*

Two old ladies travel to the mountains for vacation. "My God" complains one of them "the food here is really terrible!"

"That's right" says the other "and such small portions ..."
This describes exactly his feeling about life, said Woody Allen—and is a precise description of Anne Hedonia.

Going one step further, we run into the *psycho-vegetative depression.* Here, depressive symptoms combine with other disturbances resulting in a number of diffuse grievances in the head, stomach, heart and breathing. This is characterized by the paradoxical mixture of over-excitement, lack of peace and fear on one had and apparently endless depression on the other hand. Usually nervous exhaustion and sleep disturbances are present as well.

Sleeplessness is a real time sickness. Through too much mental activity and the use of too much nervous energy, the nerves are under too much tension so that in spite of being tired to the point of exhaustion, the necessary energy fails to let loose and sleep. St. John's wort stimulates relaxation and gives the organism a sort of "energetic kick", which activates the unconsciousness and lets one fall asleep and stay asleep.

> *Psycho-vegetative symptoms also occur in children especially in the form of bed wetting and fear at night, nervous exhaustion, concentration disturbances and stuttering.*

Depressions can occur in almost every phase of life, but especially in times of change including puberty and menopause. The typical accompanying symptoms are not only physical but also strong depressive feelings with unexplainable irritation to hysterical outbreaks, feelings of fear and worthlessness as well as difficulties in concentrating and making decisions. The simultaneous effect on the nervous and hormone system make "women's herb" a real blessing for depressions resulting from menopause as the following case makes clear:

> *A 48 year old woman who had reached menopause, suffered not only sudden outbreaks of sweat and dizziness but also deep depression. Medically, nothing could be found; she adamantly refused hormones.*
>
> *Because of the gravity of the case, St John's wort/ Hypericin was given in the form of hyperforat injections. The dosage was 5 ml every second day for one week, then 3 ml twice a week. This treatment proved very effective after three weeks. Not only did the physical grievances recede, but the woman became more open, friendly, agreeable and could go back to work.*

The Smoky Dimension

In conclusion we would like to discuss one aspect of St. John's wort, which to our knowledge has not yet been studied. A friend sent us the following story:

> In the middle of the 70's at parties and in discos, one hadn't yet heard of techno or ecstasy, but rock and grass (dried marihuana leaves) were "in" for all those who weren't against the chemical stimulation of their grey cells. I myself was very careful with all kinds of drugs and only took part among friends once—to share the experience of the others. It was a nice experience, but none that I really needed. For me the saying **"The best way to be high is to be turned on by life..."**
>
> When one is under twenty, alone, and somewhat shy, it is pleasant to have at least one cigarette at social gatherings while looking around and seeking a place to throw anchor. Tobacco was never anything for me—I assume because of my body's reaction. For this reason I got some herb tobacco once in a while from a natural food store. This mixture of dried, native plants not only burned slowly and smelled pleasant but was supposed to be healthy. One evening, as my herb tobacco supply was exhausted, I removed some of the self gathered and dried St. John's wort leaves and flowers from the hard stems and put them in my "tobacco pouch".
>
> I rolled my first cigarette. The fragrance was great— much better than the herb tobacco I had purchased! It didn't take long and I felt a transformation in myself. Suddenly the feeling of being over excited, which I had at such gatherings, disappeared. I felt centered, slightly euphoric but especially very self confident. I had to laugh about the stupid jokes. I was high—unbelievable! And it was much more intensive than I had ever experienced with "grass".

"Hey, what do you have?" my friend asked *"it smells great—can I try it?"*

"Of course" I replied.

"My word" he said *"not bad!"* With a knowing smile I gave him the St. John's wort joint.

During the following years I have permitted myself an occasional St. John's wort cigarette when I needed this soft kick. My friends also did. It became the inside tip at that time. This was the beginning of my long, great love to native herbs and their mysterious effects

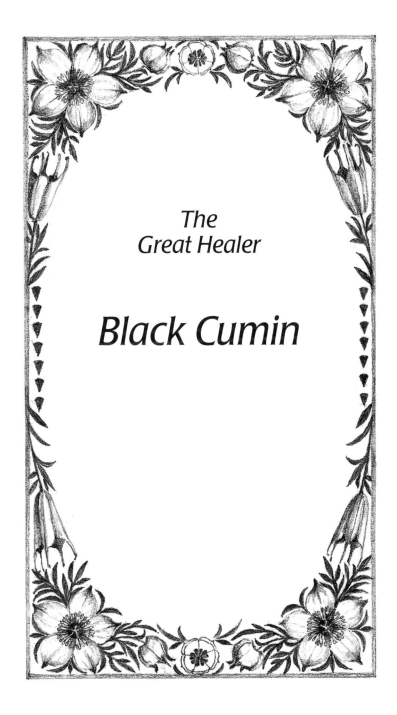

The
Great Healer

Black Cumin

After our friends heard that a new star had risen on the "hit list" of natural healing medications, we began gathering our first experiences with *Nigella sativa* from the spices in front of and behind Asiatic food stores. We quickly discovered that several very different things were offered under the name "black cumin seeds"—many couldn't be identified even today... The first spice that fit the description was declared to be "black onion seeds" and had the Indian name *Kalonji*, but the second name *Nigelle.* was a good clue. An old French name for it is *"toute épice,"* or "all-spice".

Now we were curious and as we sought further, we found black cumin seeds to be an extremely interesting spice and healing plant with as many many-sided applications as botanical species and old common names.

The Plant

Nigella sativa in a flower pot

Real, black cumin, **Nigella sativa,** is a medical plant which comes from south European, north African, and the near Orient around the Mediterranean Sea. It is sometimes listed as black cummin, black caraway, or fennel flower. From the Mediterranean lands Egypt, Syria and Turkey, it spread to Iran, Pakistan, India, and China. Hildegard von Bingen described it as a plant with "warm and dry quality."

The one year old plants which multiply by their seeds, belong to the crowfoot or buttercup family of plants *Ranunculaceae.*

They reach a height of 13 – 20 inches and appear delicate. Their stem has hairs, the leaves are divided in three. The flowers are milk-white, and in the pointed center, blue-green. They form seed capsules, which are similar to those of the poppy.

The black seeds have three sides and look very similar to onion seeds. They have given the plant its name (Latin *niger* = "black" and *nigellus* = "blackish"). They smell aromatic, more like fennel or anise than cumin, and are reminiscent of nutmeg or camphor. Their taste can be described as spicy, somewhat bitter and sharp so that they can be used as a pepper substitute. Earlier they were known as "Schwarzer Koriander" (black coriander) or "Nardensamen".

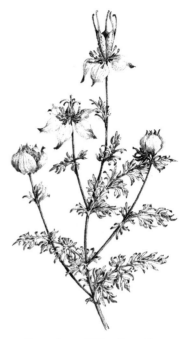

Drawing of Nigella sativa.

A rich oil with valuable contents and many-sided healing effects (more concentrated than the seeds) can be pressed from the seeds at ambient temperature. A volatile oil can also be obtained from the seeds by distillation. There are more than 20 different types, but the varieties from Egypt, Ethiopia, Sudan, Syria and Turkey are best suited for healing applications.

Other Varieties

Nigella damascena is the garden black cumin. The flower is called love-in-a-mist, (although some authors apply this name to the flower of black cumin). *Nigella damascena* also comes from southern Europe, west Asia and north

93

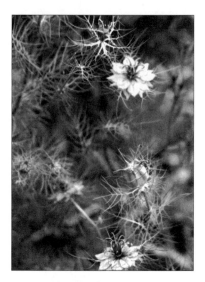

Nigella damascena in a garden

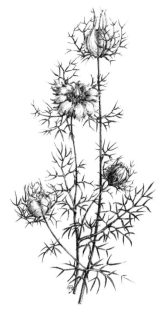

Drawing of Nigella damascena

Africa and is often called Damascus or Turkish black cumin, although the name actually refers to Syria and its capital Damascus. Since the 16th century, it has been a decorative plant "in pleasure gardens" as Hieronymus Bock mentions. Ornamental or Damascene cumin can reach 10 to 30 inches (25 – 75 cm) in height. In spite of its German nickname *Erdbeerkümmel or* "strawberry cumin", the grated seeds have a spicy smell and taste like pineapple; they are often confused with *Nigella sativa* and are also sold under that name because they are richer in oil. However, they have lower concentrations of active ingredients. Through transplantation from the far Orient to middle Europe, the plant may have changed and the healing effects may be reduced.

The finely divided leaves of ornamental cumin, which are reminiscent of fennel or dill, resemble a very fine root or hair braid in form. As a result of their impressive form and their sensitive nature, the common names are poetic such as *Jungfer in der Heck* "Virgin in the hedge" or *Gretchen im Grünen* "Gretel in the green countryside", *Braut in Haaren* "Bride in hair" or *Venushaar* "Venus hair". The latter two relate to the custom which lasted until the 18th century that the bride wore long hair decorations in order to demonstrate her virginity. Do other names such as *Blaubart* "Bluebeard" and Devil in the Bush testify to the belief that their smoke not only repels insects and poisonous animals but also witches?

Finally there is also **Nigella arvensis,** wild Nigella, which reaches a height of 4 to 8 inches (10 – 20 cm) and is compared in old herb books with the "cultivated Nigella" (*N. sativa or damascena)* as "wild Nigella". Earlier it was also called *wilder schwarzer Koriander* or "wild black coriander", *Haberkümmel* and *Roßkümmel* or "horse cumin". It was probably often confused with the black field cumin or the corn weeds, whose botanical name *Agrostémma githágo* refers to *Gith (*also *Git* or *Gitto),* the old name for black cumin seeds.

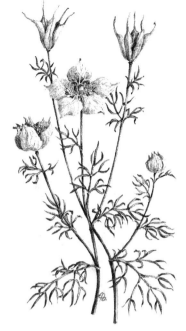

Drawing of Nigella arvensis

The Secrets of the ancient plant which was cultivated in the Orient

The oldest cultures that cultivated black cumin seeds, are those of the Egyptians and the Assyrians. The plants were used against infection and over-sensitivity (today's allergies) by the personal doctors of the pharaohs; modern research has established their effectiveness against allergic and infectious symptoms. Not only "the secret of the Pharaohs" but also that responsible for the beauty of Queen Nefertiti and Cleopatra is embodied in black cumin. It was

95

highly valued, why else was it found in the grave of Tut-
ankhamen?

Black cumin was also mentioned in the Syrian herb
book, where it had the name "black Tin-Tir," as a healing
medication applied externally for the eyes, ears and mouth,
and internally for the stomach. There are many old prescriptions for the treatment of itching, ring worm, rashes,
callouses, sores, boils—even the healing snake and scor-
pion bites when mixed with vinegar or honey and applied
to the wound.

The Copts (2 – 7th century BC), the direct descendants
of the ancient Egyptians, kept herb medicine alive and
gave it to the people of the Arabian world. In Arabic, the
seeds are called *kanün asvad* "black cumin," or *habbe
sóda,* "black seeds". One isn't surprized by the words of
the prophet Mohammed "Black cumin heals every sickness—apart from death" when one considers its broad
spectrum of application. Many Mohammedans take a few
seeds in honey every morning for strength and potency.

From southern Europe and northern Africa over Asia
Minor to India, the seeds have been traditionally used as
spice in bread and culinary dishes, where it could unfold
its digestion stimulating and gas inhibiting properties. The
bitter components make the seeds and the volatile oil effective against diarrhoea, dysentery, jaundice, gall bladder colic, congested lungs and intestinal canals, as well as
stimulating the kidneys, increasing urine excretion, aug-
menting the flow of milk, and relieving menstrual pains.
In addition, its effectiveness as a medication against worms
was known and applied especially to children.

In Indian medicine, *Nigella* is used as a spice in foods
and in the treatment of stomach cramps, diarrhoea, amoe-
bae and bacterial dysentery as well as *fluor albus* (white
vaginal excretion) and vein problems. When vision blurrs
due to infection of the mucous membrane, a special brew
from *Kalonji*, black onion seeds, curcuma (yellow spice)
and Kassumar-ginger is recommended.

The Story of Black Cumin in Middle Europe

The name *melánthion* ("black leaf") or *melásepermon* ("black seeds") for black cumin was used by Hippocrates, Dioscorides and Galen. In the first century Pliny called it *Git (Gith* also appears to be an Arabian form of the name) in his work on nature, as well as reporting a great deal about its medical advantages. In the "Hortus" of the St. Gall Cloister from 816 AD, it is listed as *Gitto* and also appears in *Capitulare* from Charlemagne as an old cultivated plant. Hildegard von Bingen called it *Githerum ratde,* and warned of its possible poisonous effects; perhaps she confused the field black caraway with the corn weed. The Latin name *Papaver nigrum* "black poppy" can also be found (in this respect it is interesting that the alkaloid Damascene which is found in Damascene cumin is said to have a narcotic effect).

Since the 16th century, black cumin, usually denoted as *Schwarzer Koriander* "black coriander", is extensively treated in all herb books. The uses known from the Orient stand in the foreground. Probably as a result of the climate, there are many prescriptions against fever, headaches resulting from the cold, toothaches, colds, congestion as well as emergency help for difficulty in breathing—which we would call bronchial asthma today. Black cumin oil was also known at this time as *Melanthium Oleum.* Prepared with sesame oil, it was used externally to prevent bed sores and to maintain clear and smooth facial skin.

Until the 18th century, black cumin was very well known among the people and used for many different things. Because of its sharp-spicy taste, it was substituted for normal caraway or pepper. Since it was often used in breads, it acquired the name *Brotwurz* "bread spice". It is hard to understand why it disappeared from our culture for almost three hundred years; in the Orient, Egypt, Syria, Turkey, India and China, it lost none of its fame.

Doesn't it sound like a tale from 1001 Nights, that after a doctor from the Nile administered it to an Arabian horse suffering from asthma, a research laboratory began studying it? Today it is on the "hit list" of natural medications and shouldn't fail in any home first aid kit.

What one should know about Cultivation

Black cumin is cultivated today primarily in the Sudan, Ethiopia, Egypt, Syria, Turkey and India. The plants grow best in warm, very sunny areas with minimal precipitation and a porous, sandy soil. The valuable contents develop best in the seed capsules under these ideal conditions.

Black cumin is an annual plant growing from September until late fall or winter. Once the flowers have bloomed and the plants begin to die from the bottom up, forcing the strength into the seed capsules (middle of summer), the seeds can be harvested. In order to avoid their taking up any dew, they are cut before sunrise and spread out to dry on large pieces of cloth. Then the capsules are threshed and the seeds brought to be pressed.

In Egypt, in accord with biological considerations, black cumin is planted in large areas of the upper Nile, and near oases in the Arabian desert. The best quality of black cumin is grown according to proven, traditional cultivation methods in Syria, south of Damascus between the Euphrates and the Tigris. In Turkey, it has been grown for many centuries in crop rotation especially in middle Anatolia and along the Aegean Sea.

Naturally the seeds contain all of the valuable components contained in the fatty oil and in the volatile oil. Apart from the fact that they have a somewhat bitter and sharp taste, one must consume a very large quantity of seeds, in order to attain the healing effect. For this reason the oil is pressed out of the seeds at ambient temperature and processed further. It is relatively viscose, has a gold-yel-

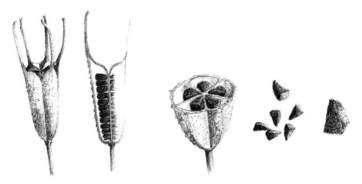

*Seed capsules (longitudinal and cross sections)
and three edged seeds (Nigella sativa)*

low color and smells very aromatic and spicy, a little like anise. For the consumer it is important that it is a native oil obtained by pressing at ambient temperature (without solvent extraction) and that the contents are not altered.

Recently, a volatile oil has also been obtained from the cumin seeds by distillation. It is thin and has a similar but more intense odor than the fatty oil.

Over one hundred Components and Active Ingredients

Black cumin works as a *complex medication;* many of its components have not yet been studied with regard to their effects or not yet discovered. The total effectiveness is a result of the synergetic effect of fatty oil, volatile oil and trace elements.

Black cumin contains about 21% protein, 38% carbohydrates and 35% plant fats and oils. More than 50% of the oils are essential fatty acids with more than one unsaturated bond. The contents of black cumin oil are similar to those of evening-primrose and borage oils, but because of its synergetic composition have a stronger effectiveness. Saponin and bitter components are among the more than 100 substances present. The amount of volatile oil is between 0.5 – 1.5%.

The high portion of unsaturated acids (with more than one double bond), such as linoleic acid and gamma linolenic acid, play a special role in the healing effect of black cumin. Modern research has shown, that these essential fatty acids, which the human body cannot synthesize, are involved in biochemical reactions which are extremely important for immune protection. Through gamma-linolenic acid, prostaglandin E1 is formed which harmonizes the entire immune system and regulates over-shooting "allergic" reactions. Prostaglandin E1 also inhibits infections and can cause an immune blockade. Gamma-linolenic acid has a stabilizing effect on the cell membrane.

Further contents of black cumin are the bitter alkaloid *Nigelline* and the glycoside *Melanthin*. Both substances stimulate the appetite, digestion and excretion. We will discuss bitter components as an important nutritional element later. Research on black cumin and the synergetic effects of its contents has not yet been completed.

The Volatile Oil

Black cumin contains 0.5 – 1.5% volatile oil with sesquiterpenes (alpha and beta pinene), sabines and sabinenhydrates, phenols (thymol and carvacrol), alcohols (1,8-cineol), terpene alcohols (borneol, linalool) and others. A particularly important component is the ethereal *nigellone semohiprepinon.* When inhaled or rubbed on the chest, it enlarges the bronchi, dissolves cramps and raises their temperature which quickly alleviates symptoms due to bronchial asthma and whooping cough. In addition nigellone inhibits release of histamine according to an Indian study, so that it might prove to be a real alternative to cortisone medication.

A further component of the ethereal oil is *thymochinon*. It inhibits infection, relieves pain, stimulates the gall bladder and works as an anti oxidant.

The Bitter Nigelline

We would like to make a few basic comments about bitter components with respect to the alkaloid component of black cumin, nigelline. (One must be careful not to confuse this with the above described ethereal component "Nigellone".)

Not only the bitter taste, but also a special energetic property belongs to this nutrient. According to the Ayurveda Theory, bitter components work cooling, light and dry; after consumption they are sharp. As a result of its regulatory effect on the fire in the body, it lowers fever, cleanses and dries excretions out. It gives tone to tissue and strengthens it, and even helps by skin irritations. It stimulates the appetite and metabolism and helps by digestive problems—for this reason bitter tonics as well as all types of cumins are famous.

Neither sour nor salty is the energetic opposite of sweet. For this reason nigelline can neutralize an excessive drive for sweets. It regulates and harmonizes all directions of taste and energetic qualities—or in today's terminology: regulates the acid-base-equilibrium. As a result of a disturbed acid-base-equilibrium due to extensive over-acidification, an ideal "milieu" for all types of infections (viral, bacterial or fungal) is formed.

It is believed that bitter components make it possible to eliminate excess acids from the body through the kidneys. In addition they have a favorable effect on the liver and the gall bladder. In the first century, Dioscorides praised the wormwood plant with the following verse:

For all that love sweets and for all
that need bitterness for the gall bladder.

Bitter components help to eliminate slime, pus and excessive fat—knowledge which the Chinese have used to reduce weight.

At a psychological level it is believed that bitter things help us to let go of old habits when they are no longer wished. This philosophy is clear in the saying "the bitter truth" and the need to change something. One must be careful of the dosage so that they don't pull together everything and lead to bitterness instead of re-establishing the total energetic equilibrium.

Black Cumin—the Secret of its Healing Power

The broad spectrum of application of black cumin shows its value as a *nutritional supplement.* Most important here is its regulating and harmonizing effect on the immune system. Its high concentration of essential, multiply unsaturated fatty acids make it effective by various disturbances of the immune system. It supports a weak immune system but can also help regulate an over-reaction.

Black Cumin for a strong Immune System

When there are too few antibodies and protective cells in the body, the immune system is weak and subject to infection. The weakened defence leads to physical and nervous-vegetative exhaustion and a tendency toward chronic afflictions or illnesses. This is the substance for cancer (or aids), since a weak immune system is not able to protect itself against transformed cells. The black cumin can even help here to dissolve "immune blockage" so that the body can carry on with the battle against a tumor.

In the opposite case, one can have an immune reaction which can be described as too strong, overshooting or even "auto-aggressive", resulting in allergic or rheumatic symptoms. The role of black cumin oil in the synthesis of prostaglandin E1 using multiply unsaturated fatty acids has already been mentioned. This substance, which resembles hormones, inhibits release of messenger substances that initiate allergies. After the first contact with an allergen (for example, by hay fever a protein from the pollen of flowers, grains or grasses), a disturbed immune system cannot discriminate between dangerous and harmless components, so that there is an over sensitivity—often for an entire lifetime. Through the harmonizing effect on the immune system, allergic reactions (which could produce symptoms such as hay fever, asthma, skin diseases, rheumatic sicknesses and food allergies) are dampened. Particularly by bronchial asthma as well as by bronchitis, coughs and congestion, the capillary broadening, cramp dissolving, and secretion dissolving effects support the immune system.

What other effects does Black Cumin Have?

Black cumin seeds have a strong anti bacterial and anti fungal effect, which helps in the fight against ineffective processes in which bacteria or fungus infection plays a role. Since black cumin seed oil stimulates bone marrow and immune cells and protects healthy cells from the damaging influence of viruses, it can inhibit tumors. Formation of the messenger substance *Interferon* cell protein, which inhibits the growth of damaging micro-organisms, is increased. Studies in the US have proved that black cumin oil destroys tumor cells, while at the same time it stimulates the bone marrow cells to increase the number of B-cells, which in turn produce antibodies. There is no damage to healthy tissue as is the case with chemical therapy. Therefore, it is useful for prevention of cancer.

Black cumin seeds support the metabolism and digestion and lower the blood sugar. For this reason it is useful in the treatment of diabetes mellitus or diabetes caused by an allergy. It is necessary that the treatment be supervised by a doctor to prevent the sugar level from sinking too far.

The Mental-Spiritual Effect

By activating the metabolism and its toning properties, black cumin is generally stimulating, for example by mental exhaustion and concentration difficulties. Vaporization of the ethereal oil in the aroma lamp, can brighten the mood when there is a tendency toward depression. The Austrian herb minister Weidinger characterizes *Nigella* as "a glance of light".

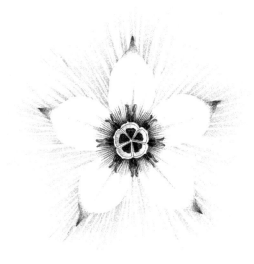

Nigella, the light flower, brightens the mood

The best Dose

In a study by a research institute in Munich, 600 allergy patients were given 500 mg of black cumin oil twice a day for three months. A clear improvement of the symptoms was observed in 85% of the patients.

These values prove that black cumin can be taken over an extended time period. Capsules (1 – 2) containing 400 mg of black cumin oil can be taken 2 – 3 times per day. The correct amount is dependent on whether they are used for prevention or treatment of acute problems. One can take 1/2 – 1 teaspoon of the oil 3 times a day. The dosage must be individually adjusted since black cumin oil increases the excretory processes quite strongly. If one insists on eating the seeds raw, the mucous membrane of the mouth and gullet can become lightly irritated.

Although neither the fatty oil nor the ethereal oil is toxic, people with a very sensitive stomach or intestine or food allergies should first try a minimal dose. The ethereal oil should only be applied to the skin in dilute form, since it can irritate it lightly.

Quality Indications versus Product-Marketing

Ideally, black cumin should come from a plantation using natural biological methods of cultivation so that the quality of the oil pressed at ambient temperature is complete and not falsified. When solvents are used for a chemical extraction this may not be the case. No oxidation, which gives it a strong taste, should have take place. The oil should be completely pure, because on the Mediterranean there are several dozen black cumin types that are not suited for healing applications.

The fact that the land of origin is "Egypt" doesn't offer any quality guarantee since real black cumin *Nigella sativa* is by no means identical with Egyptian black cumin.

The trade name "Egyptian black cumin" is sort of like a German "patent". Because of the large demand, Egypt imports more and more black cumin from Syria and Turkey so that it can be resold by product-marketing as an Egyptian ware.

THE BEST APPLICATIONS FOR BLACK CUMIN

Exact directions for use and prescriptions can be found in the appendix "Applications from A – Z"

We have seen that black cumin can be used in many different ways. By regulating a weakened or disturbed immune system, many symptoms such as infection, grippe, colds, digestion disturbances, fungus infections as well as the broad spectrum of allergic sicknesses, skin problems and rheumatic ailments can be effectively healed or at least reduced. The supportive therapy against diabetics and tumors, together with a medical treatment has been mentioned.

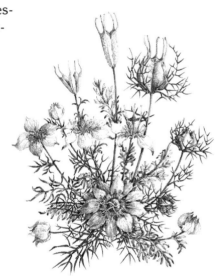

Three black cumin varieties in a small bouquet

Black cumin can be used externally and internally, as well as combining the two. We want to give you a few practical examples.

External Applications of Black Cumin

Skin Problems

By almost all infections of the skin, acne, eczema, psoriasis, skin fungus, contusions, the area can be rubbed with undiluted black cumin oil. In addition there are various prescriptions and directions for making a salve with apple vinegar and/or mud packs.

These uses are historically established. In the people's medicine, ground black cumin seeds were mixed with vinegar and laid on the area like a bandage; this was recommended to harden the sore. For treating warts and ingrown warts it was recommended to mix the seeds with urine!

For comparison we would like to give here an old prescription handed down from the Copts against itching of the skin (scabies):

Crushed black cumin seeds are cooked together with garlic, vinegar, fir resin, radish oil and soda (sodium hydroxide) and used as a salve. The degenerated skin peels away. Wash with warm water after three days.

External application of ozonized black cumin oil supported by regular internal consumption is particularly effective by chronic infected skin diseases and *neurodermitis* (skin disease with an original, nervous component). The combined treatment has a threefold effect: it stops itching, regulates the overreaction of the immune system and stimulates healing of the damaged skin. As a result of the combination of both anti allergic and infection inhibiting properties, black cumin is a real glance of light for treatment of resistant skin diseases with a nervous component.

Respiratory Illnesses

The ability of black cumin to widen capillaries, relieve cramps, and dissolve congestion is beautifully enhanced by the regulatory effect on the immune system. Bronchitis, pneumonia, stubborn coughs, festering infections of the sinuses, bronchial asthma and hay fever are alleviated by inhaling black cumin volatile oil. A few drops of the volatile oil or a cup of freshly ground black cumin seeds is placed (either in an inhalator or vaporizer) or in a bowl with a quart (1 liter) of boiling water (with a towel over the head, even if it reminds us of the horrible camomile steam baths from childhood) and inhaling for a quarter of an hour, preferably in the evening before going to sleep. The effect can be heightened by adding a little of the volatile oil (or another fragrance).

Further precautions are mentioned under internal applications. For example, regular consumption of black cumin oil capsules beginning a few months before pollen is formed, has a strong preventive effect on allergic reactions. An amazingly simple therapy for respiratory problems caused by allergic reactions, which we knew about from old sources, but apparently underestimated, was verified shortly before finishing this book:

What does black cumin have to do with the Reform of Written German?

The director of a south-western television network traveled with his crew to a meeting of various opponents of the proposed reform of written German (near Oldenburg). The couple who were supposed to play the leading roles had three cats. Immediately upon hearing of their existence and seeing the first of them, the director's eyes began to redden and his nose began to run—he was allergic to cats!

Fortunately his host knew what to do and immediately pulled out a small linen bag with black cumin seeds which had been brought back from a trip to Morocco. It came from a pharmacist versed in herbs in Marrakech, who had spread his herb treasures out before them and recommended black cumin for strong headaches, migraines, smokers cough, colds and especially for relief from hay fever and allergic asthma.

As a willing experimental rabbit, the director took the travel souvenir, rubbed the seeds and held the bag under his nose in order to breath in the volatile gases evolving from it... The effect was as astonishing for him as it was for his public; after at most a quarter of an hour, all of his problems vanished—which he verified usually required two to three weeks—and the casting could proceed without hindrance.

On the following day (by chance?) in a conversation with friends of ours, where he had his next casting, he mentioned the previous day's "key experience". In this way we learned of the wonderful connection between the anti allergic, black cumin and the written German reform.

As all-round medication "around the Head"

Many prescriptions derived from folk cures have inspired us to try them out ourselves. We would like to cite a few of the more exciting:

One of the simplest remedies for colds (and other infections of the mucous membranes such as the bronchi and wind pipe), is to burn black cumin seeds on burning coals. But they can also be crushed, moistened with distilled marjoram water, roasted in a pan, and bound in a silk or linen cloth that is held under the nose.

In order to make nose drops, the powdered seeds are mixed with old "tree oil" (olive oil). To apply, tip the head backwards as far as possible and release three drops into each side of the nose. An additional worthwhile tip: fill your mouth with water so that the oil doesn't flow back into it!

Here is one more prescription for the experienced:

Black cumin seeds and iris *roots (Iris florentina) are crushed and ground to a very fine powder. Then equal amounts of lavender blossoms, catnip, marjoram, bay leaves, and camomile are boiled and strained. Mix the liquid with the powder and use as nose drops.*

It clears the nose, the sinuses and the forehead cavity and brings the lost sense of smell again.

It used to be recommended to brush volatile oil on the inside of the nose when cataracts begin. The modern equivalent is to apply compresses with a black cumin brew for over exertion of the eyes after work with a computer monitor or reading too long.

Applying pulverised seeds to the nose is also supposed to help headaches caused by low temperatures. The same symptoms can be treated by mixing the powder with apple vinegar and when possible with "blue lily oil" (iris), and rubbing into the forehead and temples. Still another prescription for "headaches" mixes pulverized black cumin seeds with rose honey and iris oil.

For toothaches, black cumin seeds were powdered, mixed with olive oil to form a paste and painted on the tooth. Apple vinegar was also used as an additional ingredient here as well as for gargling. For (canker) sores in the mouth, black cumin seeds were chewed. These recommendations still hold today.

For earaches, black cumin seeds were baked in hot oil and the fat was applied to the ear. Today the application is easier, one drops some black cumin oil directly into the ear and massages behind the ear.

Internal Applications for Black Cumin

Commercially available black cumin oil capsules make it easy today to reduce many acute or even chronic discomforts such as avoiding pollen allergy by taking them internally. The main areas of application are:

- ❀ strengthening a weak immune system susceptible to infections
- ❀ regulation of an over shooting immune reaction by allergic illnesses
- ❀ respiratory illnesses
- ❀ stomach-intestine sicknesses
- ❀ disturbances due to hormones
- ❀ skin problems and many others

A few special prescriptions from the old treasures of experience:

The following remedy is often recommended for a repetitive fever: 2 parts black cumin seeds and 1 part parsley seeds are pulverized and taken with warm wine. One perspires and drives the fever away.

We have also found an old prescription against "bronchial asthma": The seeds are soaked in wine (or water) and removed by straining; the solution has a cleaning effect on the breast and lungs, reduces the formation of thick slime and stimulates excretion. Mornings and evenings a cup of warm solution should be drunk. It is also supposed to help when "panting and grasping for breath"! A certain amount of care must be exercised since black cumin strongly stimulates excretion, formation of urine and helps to initiate menstruation.

Inhalation with black cumin by grippe and respiratory illnesses (also of allergic types) is supported by consumption of a black cumin syrup. One portion of finely ground black cumin seeds is mixed with two portions of honey and one pressed clove of garlic. From our own experience, we understand that one might prefer a corresponding amount of grated ginger to the garlic clove. One teaspoon of this syrup is taken mornings for several weeks.

A good tea for colds can be mixed from 3 parts finely ground black cumin, 2 parts liquorice root and 1 part anise. It is brewed with hot water for 10 minutes and can be sweetened with honey.

With its broad spectrum of application, black cumin seeds prove to be an old and traditional home medication which belongs in every household first aid kit.

A few more Prescriptions

Apart from black cumin, liquorice, and anise mixtures which are not only good for colds but also relax the stomach and nerves, black cumin seeds can also be brewed alone and used to prevent intestinal gas and other digestive problems. One uses 1 teaspoon (about 1 gram) of the ground seeds per cup of boiling water. It should brew for 10 – 15 minutes and then be strained. Drink 1 cup of tea twice daily between meals.

To avoid stomach-aches, one brews a tea composed of equal amounts of black cumin, fennel and peppermint. The effectiveness is improved when a few drops of black cumin oil are added. The amount varies with individual taste. If preferred, it can also be sweetened with honey.

There is a proven recipeainst menstruation pains, especially headaches caused by hormones: 1 part finely ground black cumin seeds, 1 part pulverized anise grains and 1 part powdered cloves are mixed with one another and taken as powder. Before each meal 1 teaspoon is kept in the mouth until one can swallow it. Admittedly, one has to get used to this—but it apparently works very quickly.

The following case history is given by a middle aged woman who recognized the signals of hormone reduction and reports the effective treatment of similar symptoms:

For several years I suffered from migraine headaches with nausea and vomiting which occurred almost regularly once per month and almost always during menstruation. Therefore, one suspected a connection with the hormone system. A number of different natural healing medications did very little to reduce of the symptoms, I refused to take any "blocker".

When a therapist told me about black cumin oil and answered the question of how it works with a reference to its influence on compounds similar to hormones and the immune system, I decided to try it. I took black cumin oil in the form of capsules regularly. I always had to juggle the dosage because of the strong excretory effect and, therefore, had to use it on some days only as tea or spice.

I have no more migraines and only occasional headaches. I feel much more stable, "more immune" and look forward to the future years with their possible accompanying symptoms in a much more relaxed way than before.

Black Cumin for Skin and Body Care

Here, black cumin can look back over a long successful history, since it was used as a cosmetic by the Egyptian Queens Nefertiti and Cleopatra, who were famous for their beauty. The prescription: mix one tablespoon of black cumin oil with one tablespoon of honey and apply to the cleansed facial skin. It sounds really Oriental, doesn't it? The facial mask is allowed to work for 15 minutes and then washed it away with lukewarm water. Afterwards the skin feels smooth again—and one feels more relaxed.

Even Pliny used *nigella* and apple vinegar against skin rashes. We have included several such prescriptions using mud packs and black cumin oil in the Appendix. Treatment of eczema is supported by the internal consumption of black cumin oil capsules.

In the old herb books, black cumin oil occurs under the name *Melanthium Oleum;* it was prepared with sesame oil and used against skin blemishes and to smooth the skin. Today it is usually mixed with olive, almond or macadamia oil in order to soften the strong herb odor. When we inquired about this, we learned that there appear to be some problems in the preparation of the oil, so that relatively few commercially available products contain it.

But you can help yourself and make a *"Nigella* bran" for skin blemishes. Black cumin seeds are crushed and stirred with water. The problem areas are "rubbed" and then thoroughly washed with lukewarm water. Alternatively you can take a facial steam bath, which, by the way, also benefits the eyes.

Black cumin oil (1/2 tablespoon) can be used for damaged skin as well as to revitalize the skin in general. When the oil capsules are taken internally, the multiply unsaturated fatty acids help to remove poisons, to regenerate the intestine, and to harmonize the immune system—and all this, naturally, also benifits the beauty of the skin.

Black Cumin and Pets

Insect Repellent

For this purpose black cumin seeds, whose smoke is also reputed to drive away snakes, scorpions and even witches, is simply placed in an iron pan or directly on the hot plate and burned. To repel insects and for insect bites, black cumin oil can be directly applied together with a suitable ethereal oil such as tea tree or lavender. This also helps with sunburn.

According to old recipes, linen bags were filled with black cumin seeds and laid in the linen closet or beds. This keeps cockroaches, flees, lice and other pests away.

Animal Care

It has been common knowledge for the last few centuries not only in the Orient but also in middle Europe, that an oil, a resin and a gum extract could be obtained from black cumin which were often used against "animal sicknesses". Today 2 – 10 pounds of black cumin seeds are added to each ton of animal food. In addition to strengthening the immune system, it reduces allergic symptoms (asthma, eczema) in horses and prevents *mastitis* (udder infection) in cows.

Black Cumin Seeds in the Kitchen

We gladly admit that we have saved this chapter and the recipe section until the end because this playful use of black cumin is really fun and we are still in the middle of our creative, experimental phase.

Black Cumin as Spice

There is no botanical relationship between *Nigella sativa* and *Carum carvi,* our spice cumin, although they are used similarly. Our forefathers considered black cumin to be the more suitable "black coriander". Its spicy sharp taste made it a pepper substitute as well.

In the Arabic—and earlier even by us— the use of black cumin in baking bread was very widespread. It improves the taste of bread and at the same time makes it more easily digestible. Usually a quarter pound of crushed or ground black cumin seeds are used for two pounds of flour. It can be spread over bread or pastry together with poppy seeds..

From southwest Europe, north Africa, and west Asia, black cumin found its way to the middle East and is now cultivated in India as well. As in Turkey and other lands of the Near East, it is strewn on flat bread and used in various dishes.

The Indian name for black cumin is *kalonji*. Since it looks very similar to onion seeds, it is not only sometimes sold as "black Indian onion seeds", but also mistaken for dark Cashmere cumin *(Cuminum nigrum,* Indian *Kalajira)*. *Kalonji* is contained in many Indian spice mixtures, for example in five corn-Masala (which bears the name *Panch phoron* or "five seeds"*)* together with cumin, fennel, black mustard seed and fenugreek.

As spice, black cumin can be used instead of pepper; we fill our pepper mill with it for normal use. It is somewhat bitterer, but spicier and less sharp than pepper and gives the food a light, exotic taste. In order to make the aroma more intense, one can roast the seeds in a pan without fat before one puts them on the various dishes. Black cumin tastes especially good with *Dal,* an Indian lentil dish, and with other lentils, in pickles, chutneys, vegetables (for example, cabbage and zucchini), salads, yoghurt and quark (a milk product). A recipe follows:

Oriental cucumber salad with yoghurt sauce

Ingredients: 1 salad cucumber
1/2 pound of thick (for example Greek) Yoghurt
1/2 tablespoon of ground black cumin seeds
1 tablespoon of finely chopped fresh mint
salt

Cut the salad cucumber in thin slices and salt. Stir the mint and black cumin into the yoghurt. Add to the cucumber and mix thoroughly. Serve immediately so that the cucumber juice doesn't make the sauce watery.

A few Recipes

Chapatis—Indian flat bread
Ingredients: 1/2 pound fine, whole corn wheat or rye flour
1/2 tablespoon of finely ground black cumin
  seeds
1 tablespoon salt
3/4 cup water

Mix the flour with the spices in a bowl. Slowly add the water and knead until a smooth dough is formed. Let the dough stand for about 20 minutes. Roll the dough out to six, thin, round flat circles and bake on both sides in an iron pan.

Persian flat bread from the oven
Ingredients: 1 pound fine, whole wheat flour
1 package yeast (1 1/3 ounces)
about 6 cups lukewarm water
1/2 cup oil pressed at ambient temperature
1 tablespoon sea salt
1/2 – 1 tablespoon finely ground black cumin
  seeds

Knead the flour, yeast and water to a dough and allow to rise for 15 minutes. Add oil, salt and black cumin seeds and knead. Roll out to 4 plate sized flat circles. Put black cumin (and poppy seeds) on top and bake at about 500 degrees Fahrenheit for 10 minutes until golden brown on the upper rack of the oven.

Delicious spice slices
Ingredients: 1/2 pound of whole wheat flour
1/2 package yeast (2/3 ounce)
2 cups lukewarm water
1 tablespoon honey

Knead to a dough and allow to rise for 15 minutes. Then add the following ingredients

> 2 1/2 ounces melted butter or plant margarine
> 2 1/2 ounces ground hazel nuts or almonds
> 2 ounces honey
> 1 tablespoon cinnamon
> 1 teaspoon black cumin
> 1 pinch of ginger, cloves, nutmeg
> 1 tablespoon of powdered chocolate
> 1/2 grated lemon rind

Knead ingredients and fill a rectangular cake form. Allow to rise for another 15 minutes. Bake at 410 degrees Fahrenheit for about 1 hour in the oven.

Eat together with the following delicacy: similar to cardamom, put a pinch of black cumin in a cup of coffee. If you grind the coffee beans yourself, you can grind the black cumin seeds with them. This tastes like a fairy tale from 1001 nights, brightens the mood—and allows you to forget about a number of sicknesses.

We must admit that we also like black cumin because in addition to its therapeutic advantages, it has these marvelous uses as "nutritional supplement" for those who are completely healthy. We are none the less convinced of its unbelievable, many-sided healing applications. The experiences of past generations have veen validated by scientific experiments—such as those with St. John's wort.

The more we sought for traces of black cumin, the more clearly our plan crystallized into a comprehensive book combining primitive medicine on one hand with the newest experimental results and treatments on the other hand.*

---

* "The Healing Power of Black Cumin" by Sylvia Luetjohann, Lotus LIght, Twin Lakes 1998

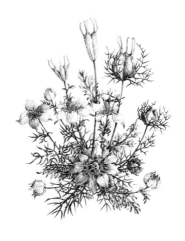

The Three Great Healers

Applications
from A – Z

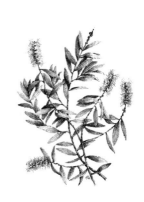

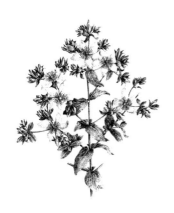

Allergies see under Asthma, bronchial, Skin Problems, and Hay fever

Anemia

St. John's wort (especially for young women)
Internally: 2 capsules or 10 drops of the fluid extract 3 times a day; after 14 days reduce to 1 capsule or 5 drops twice a day.—1 – 2 tablespoons of the freshly pressed plant juice 3 times a day, after 14 days reduce to 1 tablespoon 3 times a day.—As tea: 1 cup of St. John's wort tea sweetened with 1 tablespoon of honey 3 times a day.—Tea mixture with centaury in the ratio of 1:1.

Asthma, bronchial

Tea tree oil *Externally:* inhale the vapors from a bottle of tea tree oil or a Kleenex with several drops; Apply a compression soaked with a mixture of tea tree, eucalyptus, and thyme oils to the breast. -Mixture for the aroma lamp: tea tree oil with balm-mint and rose blossom oils.
Internally: cook 1 small onion and 2 cloves of garlic in two cups of Irish Moss Jelly for 30 minutes. Cool and press through a strainer. Mix with 1/2 cup of **red manuka** honey. Take 1 teaspoon of the syrup at a time.

St. John's wort *Internally:* Mix a pinch of aloe with the decanted tea (to thin slime).—

Middle and higher homeopathic potencies from 3 (C3 or D6 by obstructed breathing).

Black Cumin *Externally*—to be inhaled: Add 1 tablespoon of finely ground black cumin seeds (or 1/2 tablespoon of fatty- or 5 drops of ethereal black cumin oil) 1 quart (1 liter) of boiling water and inhale the warm vapors with a towel over your head.

Internally: Take 1/2 teaspoon oil or 1 capsule 2 – 3 times a day.—As tea: brew 3 parts of black cumin, 2 parts of liquorice and 1 part of anise with hot water for 10 minutes, filter and drink hot eventually sweetened with honey.—As a syrup: 1 part finely ground black cumin, 2 parts (**red manuka-**) honey and 1 crushed garlic clove or the same amount of grated ginger. Take 1 teaspoon of this syrup for several weeks.

Bed Wetting

St. John's wort (especially for nightly loss of water by small children; also by bladder catarrh)
   Internally: 1 – 2 capsules or 5 – 10 drops or 1 tablespoon of pressed juice 3 times a day.—As tea: St. John's wort pure or mixed with yarrow and horse-tails.—tea mixture of equal parts St. John's wort, yarrow and oak leaves or 2 parts St. John's wort and 1 part each of oak bark, linden blossom and bearberry (*Arctostaphylos uva ursi)* leaves. *Drink the tea early in the afternoon and then don't drink anything else*

Bladder Infection (cystitis)

(The infection is often caused by germs originating in the intestine so that it is important to treat them as well)
   Tea tree oil *Externally*—to disinfect: boil 1/2 quart (1/2 liter) water with 10 drops tea tree oil (eventually together with cajeput) and allow to cool. Wash the opening of the urinary passage with a wad of cotton wool soaked in the solution. —As bath: add 8 – 10 drops to the bath water or foot baths regularly.—Mix 3 drops with 1 teaspoon massage oil (jojoba or St. John's wort oil) and then rub the abdomen.
   Internally—by chronic bladder catarrh but not for continuous treatment: add 2 drops of tea tree oil to 1 teaspoon of **red manuka**—honey and allow to dissolve slowly in the mouth 1/2 hour before meals.

St. John's wort *Internally* -as tea: mixture with yarrow or horse-tails.—1 teaspoon of oil made with pumpkin seed oil 2 – 3 times a day.—middle homeopathic potencies 3 (C3 or D6).

Black cumin *Externally:* Rub the lower part of the stomach with black cumin oil. *Internally:* Drink a lot in general, for example black cumin tea sweetened with honey.

Bleeding, see wound treatment.

Bronchitis see under colds (infection of the respiratory system)

Colds (Infections of the Respiratory System)

Tea tree oil *Externally:* sprinkle a few drops on a Kleenex or pillowcase for a clear nose.—For Gargling: 5 – 10 drops tea tree oil in 1 glass of warm water.—To Inhale: Add 5 – 10 drops of tea tree oil (also mixed with eucalyptus or Japanese peppermint oil) in a bowl with 1 quart (1 liter) of boiling water and inhale the vapor for 10 – 15 minutes (with head under a towel). In addition to disinfect: in the aroma lamp, air moistener or vaporizer,. — Rub into breast and back, forehead and nose. As tonic for the glandular system in order to strengthen the body's defences: Mix 5 drops each of tea tree oil and lavender oil together with 1 tablespoon of jojoba oil or St. John's oil and rub into the chest and stomach, the sides of the neck, under the arms and the soles of the feet.—As bath: 5 – 10 drops in the bath water. Hot foot baths, with a few drops tea tree oil, lower fever. Otherwise rub the entire body with a washcloth soaked in water to which a few drops of tea tree oil were added (strengthens the immune system, is antiseptic, and lowers fever through perspiration).

Internally—as cough syrup: Mix 3 drops of tea tree oil with 1 tablespoon of **red manuka** honey and allow to dissolve slowly in the mouth.

St. John's oil *Internally*—as tea: St John's wort sweetened with honey (for coughs and bronchitis); Tea mixture of equal parts St. John's wort, horehound (*Marrubium*) and coltsfoot (for heavy slime); Tea mixture of 2 parts St. John's wort, 2 parts linden blossoms and 1 part peppermint (by grippe with fever).—Tincture (40%): 8 – 10 drops 2 – 3 times per day (by bronchial catarrh and asthma).

Black cumin *Externally*—To Inhale: Add 1 – 2 tablespoons of finely ground black cumin seeds (or 1/2 tablespoon of fatty oil or 5 drops volatile black cumin oil eventually together with a pressed clove of garlic) to 1 quart (1 liter) boiling water and inhale the vapor for 10 – 15 minutes with the head under a large towel). —Simplified method (for example when traveling): bind black cumin seeds in a cotton sack, rub it, and hold under the nose as needed.

Internally—as tea: Brew 1 tablespoon black cumin seeds and 1 teaspoon each of liquorice and anise with boiling water and allow to sit for 10 minutes, strain and drink sweetened with **red manuka** honey.—As syrup: Mix 1 teaspoon finely ground black cumin seeds with 1 pressed garlic clove or grated ginger and 1 tablespoon of **red manuka** honey and take 1 teaspoon several times a day.

Concentration Difficulties

Tea tree oil *Externally*—In the aroma lamp (at work): Tea tree oil with a relaxing lemon and lavender fragrance.

St. John's wort *Externally:* Rub into the forehead and temples St. John's wort oil mixed with 1 drop each of ethereal lavender and tea tree oil. *Internally*—As tea: St. John's wort and rosemary in equal portions. Further recommendations under exhaustion and nervousness

Black cumin *Internally:* 1/2 – 1 teaspoon of black cumin oil or 1 – 2 capsules 2 – 3 times per day. Powdered spice mixture: Mix 1 part each of finely ground black cumin seeds, anise and pulverized cloves. Before meals take

1 teaspoon without fluid and retain in the mouth until the powder can be swallowed. *Externally*—in the aroma lamp: use 5 drops ethereal black cumin oil mixed with lavender and a lemon fragrance.

Coughing and Hoarseness

Tea tree oil *Externally*—for gargling: 3 drops of tea tree oil, sage and thyme oil in a glass of warm water; gargle at least once a day.—To inhale: Add 10 drops of tea tree oil to a bowl with 1 quart (1 liter) hot water and inhale (with the head under a large towel). Before going to bed put a few drops of tea tree oil on the pillowcase.—To massage: Rub a mixture of tea tree oil or a mixture of 10 drops each of tea tree oil and pine needle oil (**red manuka and white manuka,** if available) together with 50 ml (1/2 cup of St John's wort oil) into the breast and back (kidneys!); In addition to the breast and kidney area also massage gently into the lymph glands on the sides of the neck and under the arms as well as into the bottoms of the feet.

Internally: When you have a persevering cough (only occasionally) drop 3 drops of tea tree oil on 1 tablespoon of **red manuka** honey and allow to dissolve slowly in the mouth.

St John's wort *Internally*—as tea: St John's wort sweetened with Honey (dissolves slime).

Black cumin *Externally:* 1 – 2 tablespoons of black cumin seeds or 1/2 tablespoon black cumin oil in a bowl with 1 quart (1 liter) of boiling water and inhale the vapors for 10 – 15 minutes (with head under a large towel).—Simplified method (for Example when travelling): bind black cumin seeds in a cotton sack, rub on it and hold under the nose as needed.

Internally—as tea: brew 3 parts black cumin, 2 parts liquorice and 1 part anise with boiling water for 10 minutes, sweeten with **manuka** honey and drink.—As syrup: Mix 1 part finely ground black cumin seeds and 1 pressed clove of garlic or the same amount of grated ginger with 2 parts **manuka** honey. Take 1 teaspoon of this syrup mornings for an extended period.

Contussions, See under wound treatment.

Depression

St. John's wort (also by winter depression, panic and in connection with menopause) *Internally:* Take 1 – 2 capsules or 20 – 30 drops of the fluid extract or 1 – 2 tablespoons of the pressed plant juice 3 times a day; reduce to half the dosage after 14 days. It is necessary to take for a long period!—Middle homeopathy potency 3 (C3 or D6) for a longer period.—As tea: 3 parts St. John's wort tea and 2 parts balm-mint and 1 part marjoram (for nervousness combined with depression); Equal portions of St. John's wort, balm-mint, valerian and passion flower (menopause).

Diabetes

Tea tree oil *Externally*—For treatment of diabetic gangrene (death of skin tissue due to diabetes): Mix tea tre oil with massage oil and rub into the afflicted area.

    Black cumin *Internally*—Lower blood sugar levels and allergic factors (by strengthening the immune system): Take 1 – 2 oil capsules or 1/2 teaspoon oil 3 times a day for a longer period. *Important: A doctor's control is absolutely necessary to avoid lowering the sugar level too far.*

Diarrhoe, see under stomach and intestine illnesses.

Earaches

Tea tree oil *Only externally:* Mix a few drops of tea tree oil with 1 egg holder (about 1 tablespoon of warm olive oil and dab into the ear canal with a Q-tip. Never use undiluted! By long lasting aches soak some cotton wool in the mixture and place in the ear canal. Rub some tea tree oil diluted with a carrier oil behind the ear.

Black cumin *Only externally:* Drop a few drops of black cumin oil directly into the ear canal and massage some oil behind the ear.—Or: bake the black cumin seeds in heated black cumin oil and peel. Paint this brew in the ear.

Exhaustion, Vegetative

Tea tree oil *Only externally:* Add 5 drops of tea tree oil and 5 drops of lavender oil to bath water. It builds one up and relaxes.

St. Johns's wort *Internally:* Take 1 – 2 capsules or 10 – 15 drops of tincture or 1 tablespoon of fresh pressed plant juice, for several weeks.—As tea: St. John's wort as "single drug" or tea mixture of 2 parts St. John's wort, 2 parts balm-mint and 1 part rosemary (for exhaustion and over working). Super nerve tea: St. John's wort, goldenrod and balm-mint in equal portions.

Internally (to stabilize the immune system): Take 1 – 2 capsules or 1/2 teaspoon 2 –3 times a day.

Eye Soreness

Black cumin *Externally*—As eye compress: After too much exertion of the eyes for example, from a computer monitor, television or prolonged reading, boil 1 tablespoon of black cumin seeds in 1 cup of water and allow to sit for 10 minutes. Pour through a strainer. Soak two wads of cotton wool

in the solution and lay them on the eyes for 10 minutes. —
Rub the temples with black cumin oil before going to sleep.

Flatulence, gas accumulation

St. John's wort *Internally:* Take 1 – 2 tablespoons of
pressed plant juice 3 times a day for 14 days.—As tea:
St. John's wort with fennel and anise in equal portions. —
St. John's wort oil made yourself with black cumin oil: take
1 teaspoon as needed 2 – 3 times a day.

Black cumin *Externally*—as compression: apply compression soaked with apple vinegar and black cumin to the
stomach.

Internally—as tea: make a tea of equal parts black cumin, fennel and peppermint. Add 3 – 7 drops of black cumin oil. It can be sweetened with honey.— By terrible
discomfort—as tonic: Boil 2 parts apple vinegar with 1 part
finely ground black cumin seeds, and then add 1 part black
cumin oil. Take 1 tablespoon before meals 3 times a day.

Fungus Infection

Tea tree oil *Only externally*
Fungus in the mouth: Gargle or paint the mouth cavity
with diluted tea tree oil.

Use only controled biological quality with low concentrations of toxic cineol.

Skin and foot fungus: After thoroughly washing and
drying the area, apply tea tree oil twice a day (also possible with diluted solution).

Vaginal fungus: Place a tampon soaked with tea tree
oil in the vagina.—For washing the vagina mix 20 – 30
drops of tea tree oil (to distribute throughout the water add
warm milk as emulgator) in 1/2 quart (1 liter) of warm
distilled water.

By suspicion of *Candida* infection (also in the intestine) add 1 teaspoon of tee tree oil to the bath water and gargle with 3 drops of tea tree oil in 1/2 glass of warm water regularly.

Be careful to use a good controled biological quality with low concentrations of toxic cineol.

See under *Vagina, Infection of*

Black cumin *Externally* (for skin fungus): Stir 2 parts apple vinegar with 1 part finely ground black cumin seeds and 1 part mud packs (or starch). Apply twice a day to the afflicted skin area.

Internally: Cook 2 parts apple vinegar with 1 part very fine black cumin seeds and 1 part black cumin oil to a syrup consistency and take 1 tablespoon before meals 3 times a day.

Grippe See colds and infections of the respiratory system.

Gall and Liver Diseases

St. John's wort *Internally*—St. John's wort oil: For gall attack take 2 – 3 teaspoons daily.—As tea: Drink 2 – 3 cups of St. John's tea daily (by tendency to gall attacks); Mix St John's wort and aloe in the ratio of 1:1 (as liver/gall tea); Tee mixture of St. John's wort, yarrow, horsetail (*Equisetum)*, and chicory (with root) in equal portions (by gall stones). For the liver: Take 1 cup St. John's wort alone or in combination with swallowwort and gentian (prophylactic); Mixture of St. John's wort and yarrow (stimulating); mixture of St. John's wort, wormwood, and sage (strengthening).

Black Cumin (to increase gall bladder secretion) *Internally:* Take 2 – 3 teaspoons black cumin oil or drink 2 – 3 cups of tea from back cumin seeds.

Grippe infect see under colds (and infections of the respiratory system)

Hay Fever

Tea tree oil *Externally*—To inhale: Make a mixture of 40 drops tea tree oil (and if available 20 drops of **red manuka** and **white manuka** oil) with 20 drops of cypress and 20 drops of cedar oil. Add 5 – 8 drops of this mixture to a bowl with hot water or an aroma lamp.

Internally: Allow 1 drop of tea tree in **red manuka** honey to dissolve in the mouth. Take as a syrup twice a day for a maximum of 14 days.

Black cumin *Externally*: Add 1 – 2 tablespoons of black cumin seeds or 1/2 tablespoon of black cumin oil to a bowl of hot water. Inhale the vapors several times a day (with the head under a large towel). Simplified version (for traveling): Bind black cumin seeds in a cotton sack, rub it when needed and hold under the nose.

Internally: As preventative begin taking black cumin (1 capsule or 1/2 teaspoon oil 2 – 3 times a day) a few months before pollen is released and continue until spring/summer. During the pollen release take 1 – 2 capsules or a maximum of 2 teaspoons of the oil 2 – 3 times a day as the maximal dose.

Headaches

Tea tree oil *Externally:* Coat the temples with tea tree oil and lavender oil eventually diluted with water. Mix with St. John's wort oil and gently massage into the neck.—Aroma lamp: Mixture of 5 drops tea tree oil with 3 drops lavender and 1 drop each of ethereal lemon and muscatel sage oil.

St. John's wort (especially for headaches caused by nervousness or hormonal imbalance)

Externally: Rub St. John's wort oil softly into the temples and neck, eventually with a few drops of tea tree oil and lavender oil. *Internally:* Take 1 – 2 capsules or 5 – 10 drops of the fluid extract or 1 – 2 tablespoons of the freshly pressed juice. Very effectively alternated with black cumin oil. —As tea: St John's wort pure or in a mixture with blessed thistle (*Cnicus benedictus*).

Black cumin *Only internally*

(especially by headaches caused by hormones and migraines): Mix 1 part finely ground black cumin seeds, 1 part finely ground anise seeds and 1 part powdered cloves. Take 1 teaspoon of the mixture before meals and keep in the mouth until the powder can be swallowed (do not take with water!).—For long term treatment and adjustment of the hormone system take 1 – 2 capsules or 1/2 teaspoon of oil 2 – 3 times daily.

Heart problems due to Nervousness

St. John's wort *Internally:* Take 1 – 2 capsules or 5 – 10 drops of tincture or 1 – 2 tablespoons of the fresh pressed juice 3 times a day in the afternoon and evening.—As tea: St John's wort pure or in a mixture with balm-mint or hawthorn or mistletoe.—Middle homeopathic potencies 3 (C3 or D6). —By heart problems originating in the stomach (gastro-cardio symptom complex): Take 6 – 8 drops of the fluid extract with sugar or water.

Haemorrhoids

Tea tree oil *Externally*—Rub in undiluted or mix with some oil. Special recipe: mix 4 drops of tea tree oil or **white manuka** oil and 4 drops of cypress oil with 10 ml of St. John's wort oil. —As bath: Add 10 drops of tea tree oil to a warm bath in sitting.

St. John's wort *Externally:* Dab with the mother liquid (or homeopathic D 1 potency) carefully. *Internally:* Drink 1 liquor glass of St. John's wort tincture (3 handfuls of fresh blossoms in 1/2 quart (1/2 liter) liquor).

Black cumin *Externally:* Burn black cumin seeds in an iron pan or directly on the oven plate to *black cumin ashes.* Apply either alone or mixed in a ratio of 1:1 with black cumin oil to the haemorrhoids. —As bath sitting: 15 ml black cumin oil in 1 quart (1 liter) water.

Immune System, Strengthening of

(By general susceptibility, acute and preventative, as well as by stress due to monitor radiation and computer work).

Tea tree oil *Only externally*

Bath: A warm bath with 8 – 10 drops of tea tree oil added twice a week.

Massage: Rub tea tree massage oil diluted to 5% over the entire body once a week or rub the hand surfaces and foot soles strongly every day.

1. Recipe for lymph gland tonic: 10 drops of tea tree oil or mix 5 drops each of tea tree oil and lavender oil with 1 tablespoon (10 ml) of skin oil. Rub the juice into the lymph glands on the neck gently.
2. Recipe: Mix 7 drops each of tea tree oil, lavender and bergamot oil as well as 4 drops of sandalwood with 1/2 cup (50 ml) St John's wort oil. Very good to rub into the lymph glands on the throat of the neck, the upper breast and the solar plexus to the groins.

Aroma lamp: burn a mixture of tea tree oil with, for example, lavender, bergamot, and sandalwood oil.

European "Maori-mixture": In so far as one can find **red manuka** and **white manuka** oil, mix with lavender or a lemon oil and add to a massage oil or vaporize in an aroma lamp.

Black cumin *Externally*—to inhale: 1/2 tablespoon fatty black cumin oil (or 5 drops of volatile oil in a quart (1 liter) of water twice a day —As bath: Add 1/2 tablespoon fatty or 5 – 8 drops ethereal black cumin oil with 1 tablespoon cream (as emulgator) and add to bath water.—As massage: Mix

15 – 20 drops ethereal black cumin oil with 1 cup (100 ml) skin oil or body lotion.

Internally: Take 1 – 2 capsules or 1/2 – 1 teaspoon black cumin oil 2 – 3 times per day.

Infections

Tea tree oil *Externally:* As addition to compressions.

St. John's wort *Externally:* St. John's wort for wound compressions and ointment bandages. *Internally* (by mucus membrane infections, for example of the stomach, uterus and vagina): Middle homeopathic potency 3 (C3 or D6)

See also under skin problems and wounds.

Intestine fungus see fungus infections.

Intestine Parasites

(For example worms, flagellata, intestinal and liver leeches which cause many problems some of which are very diffuse)

St. John's wort (Worm remedy) *Externally:* Rub the area around the belly button with St. John's wort oil (especially effective by small children). *Internally:* take l teaspoon St. John's wort oil 3 times a day. To avoid possible constipation combine with wormwood tincture (vermouth).

Black cumin *Internally:* Take oil capsules regularly 3 times a day. Boil: 2 parts apple vinegar with 1 part finely ground black cumin seeds and 1 part black cumin oil, until a syrup-like consistency is reached. Take 1 tablespoon 3 times a day before meals.

Intestinal fungus see fungus infections.

Kidney Problems

St. John's wort *Internally*—against kidney stones: Take mornings on an empty stomach 1 – 2 teaspoons of St. John's wort oil (made with pumpkin seed oil) for 14 days from full moon onwards by a diminishing moon, after the new moon make a 14 day pause.—Kidney tea: take 2 – 3 cups of St. John's wort daily pure or in the ratio of 1:1 with yarrow or horsetail (also over a longer period or as a preventative).

Black cumin *Externally:* Apply a kidney compression with finely ground black cumin seeds mixed with warm olive oil.

Internally: Mix 1 teaspoon of finely ground black cumin seeds (or 1/2 teaspoon oil), 1 pressed garlic clove with 2 tablespoons of honey. Take 1 teaspoon before meals.

Menstrual Cramps

St. John's wort *Externally:* For cramp-like menstruation pains in the stomach, rub St. John's wort oil gently in or apply compressions. *Internally:* About 1 week before the normal period, begin taking capsules or fluid extract as a preventative.—As tea: St. John's wort pure or by weak bleeding mixed in equal portions with Lady's mantle (*Alchemilla vulgaris*) or yarrow or wild vermouth (*Artemisia vulgaris*).—For painful menstruation take together or alternating with mistletoe tea; or St. John's wort mixed with equal portions of hawthorn (*Marrubium*), centaury, thyme and hyssop.—By too heavy menstruation (to lesson bleeding): St. John's wort and yarrow.—For bleeding in menopause: Tea from St. John's wort and mistletoe.

Tea tree oil *Only Externally*

Antiseptic mouth wash: 2 – 3 drops of tea tree oil mixed with some camomile oil and dissolve in warm water; use several times a day.—Add 3 drops of tea tree oil and 1 drop of Japanese peppermint oil and 1 drop of thyme oil in some warm milk and then dilute with 1/2 glass of warm water.

Mouth sores (also for mouth odor): Gargle with 3 – 5 drops of tea tree oil in warm water 2 – 3 times a day. To disinfect place a few drops directly on your tooth brush.

Lip sores (from Herpes-virus): Dab the blisters with pure oil 3 times a day, use Q-tips by danger of infection.

Fungus in mouth: Paint dilute tea tree oil directly in the mouth cavity or gargle.

Here one must pay particular attention to controled biological quality without worrying about the cineol which is toxic at high concentrations.

St. John's wort *Externally:* By infection of the mucous membrane of the mouth gargle with a diluted St. John's wort tincture. *Internally:* Homeopathic low potency mother solution diluted to 10% (D1).

Black cumin *Only externally*

Rub the mouth cavity with black cumin oil (afterwards spit the oil out)

Muscle and Joint Pains

Tea tree oil *Externally*—as massage: Tea tree oil mixed with some skin oil (for example warm almond, jojoba or St. John's wort oil), by acute or chronic infection of the joints rub deep into the painful areas. For a small supply: Use 30 drops of oil with 50 ml carrier oil. Tea tree oil can be mixed with lavender, marjoram or rosemary oil. —As bath: 8 – 10 drops added to the bath water.

St. John's wort *External*—St. John's wort oil made with hemp-oil for rubbing in (also by torn muscles, and contusions, sprains and tension in the back)

Black cumin oil *External:* Massage the painful areas with warm black cumin oil twice a day. See also wound treatment.

Nervousness

St. John's wort *Internally:* By disturbance of the nervous equilibrium take 1 – 2 capsules or 10 – 15 drops of the tincture or 10 – 15 drops of St. John's wort oil or 1 tablespoon of freshly pressed plant juice 2 – 3 times a day for several weeks.—Middle homeopathic potency 3 (C3 or D6).—As tea: 1 cup of St. John's wort tea sweetened with 1 tablespoon of honey before going to sleep.—Super nerve tea (to relax): St John's wort, goldenrod and balm-mint. —Tea to strengthen nerves (after overworking and by exhaustion): Mixture of 2 parts St. John's wort and balm-mint and 1 part rosemary.

See also *Depression.*

Neuralgia (Nerve Pains)

(Nerve infections; *trigeminus,* migraines, slipped disk, coccyx neuralgia; paralysis and numb feelings)

External: Especially face neuralgia and nerve pains in the back, arms and legs, rub in St. John's wort (made with sesame oil).—Original tincture, also alternating with arnica tincture or salve.

Internal: Take 1 tablespoon of fresh pressed plant juice diluted with water or camomile tea several times a day.

By trigeminus neuralgia: Rub the skin area regularly with St. John's wort oil, supported by taking St. John's wort tea over an extended period.

by post traumatic processes after injury and damage to nerves through dreams: Low to middle homeopathic potencies 1 – 3 (C1 – C3 or D1 – D6).

Nose and Sinuses (rhinitis and sinusitis)

Tea tree oil *Only externally*
Clogged nose and sinusitis: 5 – 10 drops of tea tree oil in a bowl with 1 quart (1 liter) hot water and inhale the vapors for 15 minutes (with the head under a large towel).— By sinusitis rub tea tree oil undiluted into the skin of the temples, the nose and the cheeks.

Add 8 – 10 drops of tea tree oil to the bath water as well as (in combination with eucalyptus oil, peppermint oil and niaouli oil) in the aroma lamp.

Sores of the mucous membrane of the nose: Inhale warm vapors or apply tea tree oil directly with a Q-tip.

Black cumin *Externally:* Brew 1 – 2 tablespoons of black cumin seeds or 1/2 tablespoon of black cumin oil with 1 quart (1 liter) of boiling water and inhale the hot vapors for 15 minutes (with the head under a large towel). Extremely effective since the secretion is dissolved.—Simplified method (for travel): Bind black cumin seeds in a sack, rub and hold under the nose as needed.

Internally: Support external treatment by taking black cumin tea and oil capsules.

Poisoning

Black cumin *Internally*—to reduce vomiting: Decant tea from 1 tablespoon of black cumin seeds and add 1 teaspoon cloves, drink unsweetened. By continued vomiting take 1 oil capsule or 1/2 teaspoon oil.

Tea tree oil *Only externally:* Mix a few drops of tea tree oil with a good carrier oil pressed at ambient temperature and warm; particularly suitable is St. John's wort oil. Apply to the painful body areas. It increases the mobility. Lavender, marjoram and rosemary oils also have a favorable effect.—As bath: Add to the bath water 8 – 10 drops of tea tree oil mixed with lavender for relaxation.—As compression: place a cloth in warm water, wring, drop a few drops of tea tree oil on it, and lay over the painful area.

St. John's wort *Only externally:* Use St. John's wort oil for massage; eventually tea tree oil (see above) and other ethereal oils. -Salve mixture: St. John's wort and aloe.

Skin Problems

Tea tree oil *Only Externally*
Acne/pimples: Apply tea tree oil undiluted (or in dilute form) to the skin area with finger or Q-tips 3 – 4 times on the 1st day. In the following days repeat 2 – 3 times. For washing take 3 – 6 drops in warm water. In addition use a tea tree soap and an antiseptic non fat skin cream or moisture lotion with tea tree oil or make your own product with a few drops of tea tree oil.

Furuncles and Abscesses: Clean the skin area carefully and coat with tea tree oil 2 – 3 times per day to disinfect even when in an open condition. As compress: Mix tea tree oil with warm water, soak a piece of gauze in the solution and lay over the furuncles for several hours.—As healing compression: mix tea tree oil with warm water, soak a cloth in it and lay over the boil for several hours.—Mud packs, apply clay poultice with some warm water mixed with a few drops of tea tree oil to the afflicted area and rinse after 1/2 – 1 hour.

Skin Eczema: Apply in accordance with experience (test!) undiluted or in ratio 1:10 with a high quality skin cream (almond, jojoba).

Neurodermitis: Apply undiluted if possible. Otherwise do not mix with a fatty body oil but add some milk and then dilute with water. (By this "multiple allergy, tea tree oil reduces itching which in turn reduces the scratching and the danger of further infection).

Psoriasis (scaly patches): Mix 10 drops each of tea tree oil, cajeput oil and myrrh oil with 1 cup (100 ml) of a good skin oil or mix 10 drops each of **red manuka oil,** lavender oil and bergamot oil with 1 cup (100 ml) of carrier oil. Rub in twice a day.

Herpes (blister rash): Apply tea tree oil directly to the blisters. Use Q-tips if there is particular danger of infection.

Skin fungus (thrush and Candida): Apply tea tree oil or a diluted solution to the washed area twice a day.

St John's wort
Externally

By blemished, flaky skin: Dab St. John's wort tincture on the afflicted skin area and/or rub in St. John's wort oil. Volatile tea tree oil or lavender oil can be used very well with it. It is also suitable for the final treatment of acne and seborrhoea.

For sores (for example from lying in bed): A good combination is St. John's wort with arnica and marigolds (also commercially available in salves).

Boils and abscesses: Massage St. John's wort carefully into the tissue.

Itching rashes (psoriasis): Treat with St. John's wort oil or tincture in accordance with compatibility.

Eczema (reddening of the skin) and sunburn: Rub St. John's wort oil into the skin area. The strong reddening disappears quickly. Stay out of the sun!

Herpes (blister rash) as well as Herpes zoster (shingles):
Dab carefully with St. John's wort oil or a strongly diluted tincture. Cover blisters with oil soaked compressions.
Internally
By infectious and allergic skin problems, psoriasis and Herpes: Use homeopathic potencies from 3 (C3 or D6) and higher.

Black cumin
Externally
Acne, skin rashes due to nervousness, eczema, skin fungus etc.
1. Mix 1 part powdered black cumin seeds with 2 parts of apple vinegar and allow to stand for 6 hours. Filter and again allow to stand for 24 hours. Decant the fluid and mix the residue with black cumin oil in the ratio of 1:1. Apply several times a day.
2. Extend the above recipe by mixing 4 parts of the residue with 2 parts of healing earth and 1 part apple vinegar. Heat for 2 – 3 minutes stirring constantly. Just before applying to the skin (preferably over night), mix with black cumin oil in a ratio of 1:1.
3. Heat 2 parts apple vinegar with 1 part powdered black cumin seeds and thicken with 1 part corn or potato starch. Apply several times a day.

If the skin is compatible (by skin allergies) with the fatty oil, pure black cumin oil can be carefully massaged into the skin.
Face steam baths: Pour 1 quart (1 liter) of hot water over 1 – 2 tablespoons of black cumin seeds (or 1/2 tablespoons fatty oil or 5 drops volatile black cumin oil) in a bowl and allow the steam and gaseous components to work on the face. Repeat at least once a day.
Internally
By eczema and neurodermitis: Take 1 – 2 capsules or 1/2 teaspoon black cumin oil 2 – 3 times a day.

Sleep Disturbance

Tea tree oil /red manuka *Externally*: Mix 2 drops of tea tree oil or red manuka oil and 5 drops of lavender oil with 1 tablespoon (10 ml) St. John's wort oil and massage the loins and stomach area with it before going to sleep.

Internally: Mix together 2 parts apple vinegar, 2 parts red manuka honey and 1 cup of water and drink 1/4 cup before going to bed.

St. John's wort *Internally*—as tea: 2 – 3 cups of St. John's wort over the day or 1 cup sweetened with honey before going to bed.—Super tea mixture for sleeping: St. John's wort, valerian root and hops in equal portions; or 2 parts St. John's wort, 2 parts valerian and 1 part lavender (to improve the taste).—Further recommendations (capsules, drops, pressed plant juice or homeopathic potency 3 (C3 or D6) as indicated under "Nervousness".

Sore Throat (Angina)

Tea tree oil *Externally*: Gargle thoroughly with 5 drops in 1 glass of warm water 2 times each day, also for prevention.

Internally: Add 3 drops to 1 teaspoon **red manuka** honey and allow to dissolve slowly in the mouth; as addition to juices from citrus fruits (with high vitamin C content).

Stomach and Intestine Problems

St. John's wort
(For a nervous, irritated stomach-intestinal catarrh, stomach membrane infection and ulcers)

Externally: For stomach-aches rub the entire area of the solar plexus gently with St. John's wort oil.

Internally: Make St. John's wort oil using black cumin oil: Take 5 – 10 drops of St. John's wort oil pure or (with children) in 1 tablespoon of milk or dropped onto some sugar for stomach-aches. For colics and cramps raise the dose to 2 – 3 teaspoons per day.—For a nervous stomach-intestinal disturbance: Take a few drops of St. John's wort oil in 1 teaspoon of honey every morning and swallow with saliva. As tincture (50%): 8 – 10 drops 2 – 3 times per day. For the same indications 1 – 2 tablespoons of freshly pressed juice 3 times a day for 14 days is recommended. —As tea: Drink 1 cup St. John's wort tea before every meal. By a nervous stomach with diarrhoea: St. John's wort and yarrow in the ratio of 1:1. For swelling and gas: St. John's wort, fennel and anise. To strengthen the stomach: St. John's wort, wormwood and sage or centaury.

Black cumin

Externally: Mornings and evenings a warm to hot stomach compression soaked with a mixture of pulverized black cumin seeds (or a few drops of black cumin oil) and apple vinegar.

Internally: Mornings and evenings take 1 tablespoon of black cumin seeds or some oil.

—For heartburn, stuffed feeling, diarrhoea and constipation: Stir 2 teaspoons of black cumin oil in a cup with warm milk and sweetened with 1 tablespoon of honey.

Toothaches and Gingivitis

Tea tree oil *Only externally*
Tooth infection and bacterial tooth deposit: Gargle with 3 – 5 drops of tea tree oil in 1/3 glass of warm water.— Rub tea tree oil directly into the gums.—Add a few drops of tea tree oil to disinfect the toothbrush.

Toothaches and gum bleeding (also after dental treatment): mix 2 – 3 drops of tea tree oil with some camomile oil and add to warm water. Use 3 times a day as an anti-septic mouth wash. Works to lessen pain antibacterially.

Mouth sores: Mix thoroughly 1/4 cup lemon juice with 1/4 cup **red manuka** honey.

Take 1 teaspoon as needed.

St. John's wort *Only externally*

For prevention of cavities, gum infection and recession: Use toothpaste with hypericum oil.

Black cumin *Externally:* Boil 1 glass apple vinegar with 2 tablespoons finely ground black cumin seeds. Strain. Rinse the mouth with it for several days.—Rub painful area with 1 – 2 drops of oil.

Internally: Mix finely ground black cumin, anise seeds and cloves in equal portions. Allow the powdered mixture to gather saliva in the mouth until it can be swallowed.

Tumors

Black cumin (Cancer preventative by stimulating bone marrow cells with destruction of micro-organisms and tumor cells) *Internally:* 1 – 2 capsules black cumin oil 2 – 3 times daily over an extended period.

Vagina Infection

(Infections can be caused by fungus infection, bacteria or parasites, although the treatment remains largely the same.)

Tea tree oil *Only externally*

Do not wash the vagina region with soap but add a few drops of tea tree oil to the water.

Vagina (outer portion) wash or tampon: Add 10 drops of tea tree oil to a little warm milk, shake well with 1/2 quart (1/2 liter) purified or distilled water and make a vagina wash with this mixture or soak a tampon in it and insert in the outer portion of the vagina.

Dose for a vagina (internal) wash: 1/2 tablespoon (5 ml) tea tree oil in 1/2 quart (1 liter) water. It may prickle slightly but it must not burn.

Bath sitting: Add 10 drops of tea tree oil to the bath water.

Massage: Mix 10 drops of tea tree oil, 10 drops of lavender and muscatel laurel with 50 ml St. John's wort oil. Massage once a day into the outer vagina.

Black cumin *Only externally:* Clean the outer vagina with highly dilute ethereal black cumin oil (5 drops in 2 quarts (2 liters) of water) or take a bath sitting.

"Aroma tampon": Mix 10 drops of ethereal black cumin oil with 30 ml jojoba oil. Soak the tampon in it and insert; change several times a day.

Varicose Vein Sores

Tea tree oil *Only externally:* bathe the open wound with warm water to which a few drops of tea tree oil (eventually mixed with milk or cream as emulgator). Wrap the leg with a compression, soaked with a mixture of 3 parts olive oil and 1 part tea tree oil. This heals quickly.—As preventive, apply a lotion containing 10% tea tree oil (this is about 20 drops of tee tree oil in 1 tablespoon of moisturizing lotion).

Black cumin *Only External:* Heat black cumin seeds in an iron pan and stir with orpine to a paste. Apply to the well cleaned legs and after drying, wrap with a sterilized bandage. Renew 1 or 2 times a day.

Wound Treatment

Tea tree oil *Only externally*

By contusions (relieves pain, reduces swelling, and speeds healing): Put a few drops of tea tree oil directly on the contusion. —As compression: Dunk a cloth in cold water, wring thoroughly and sprinkle with 3 – 5 drops of tea tree oil. Apply the compression.

By open wounds, cuts and scrapes (works disinfecting, antiseptic and relieves pain): Apply tea tree oil directly or in a dilution of 1:10 with almond oil.—Wash with a 10% tea tree oil lotion and apply a bandage soaked with it (heals quicker).—Compression: Mix some healing earth with water and a few drops of tea tree oil. Spread over the wound and cover with a gauze bandage (works antiseptic and heals quicker).

St. John's wort *Externally*

By blows, punctures, cuts, burns, bleeding wounds, contusions, and bruises (especially in areas with a lot of nerves): Apply compressions soaked in St. John's wort oil. Change several times a day.

Especially by burns: Make St. John's wort oil with linseed oil.

Additional disinfection: Alcoholic tincture (50%) or use liquid homeopathic D1 solution. Reduces blood flow.

Poorly healed wounds and sores: Tincture or salves, good combined with arnica.

Wound area (For example due to lying too long on one side): A very good combination of St. John's wort with arnica and marigolds (also in commercially available salve mixtures).

Internally

By post traumatic processes after injury, nerve damage due to trauma/shock and for wound treatment by destruction of nerve endings: Low to middle homeopathic potencies 1 – 3 (C1 – C3 or D1 – D6) as "arnica of the nerves".

Black cumin *only externally:* Apply black cumin oil directly or mixed with apple vinegar to the wound.

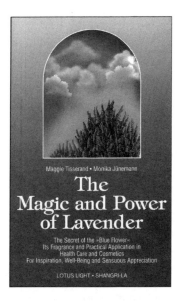

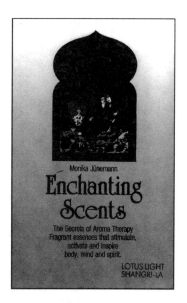

Magie Tisserand · Monika
Jünemann

The Magic and Power of Lavender

The Secret of the Blue Flower

The scent of lavender practically has permeated whole regions of Europe, contributing to their special character, and dominated perfumery for most of its history. To this very day, lavender has remained one of the most familiar, popular, and utilized of all fragrances.

This book introduces you to the delightful and enticing secrets of this plant and its essence, demonstrating its healing power, while also presenting the places and people involved in its cultivation. The authors have asked doctors, holistic health practitioners, chemists, and perfumers about their experiences and share them – together with their own with you.

136 pages, $ 9.95
ISBN 0-941524-88-4

Monika Jünemann

Enchanting Scents

The Secrets of Aromatherapy
Fragrant Essences that Stimulate, Activate and Inspire Body, Mind and Spirit

Today we are just as captivated by the magic of lovely scents and as irresistably moved by them as ever. The effects that essential oils have can vary greatly. This book particularly treats their subtle influences, but also presents and describes the plants from which they are obtained. It beckons you to enter the realm of sensual experience and journey into the world of fragrance through essences. It is an invitation to use personal scents to activate body and spirit. Here is a key that will open your senses to the limitless possibilities of benefitting from fragrances as stimulants, sources of energy, and means of healing.

128 pages, $ 9.95
ISBN 0-941524-36-1

Sources of Supply:

The following companies have an extensive selection of useful products and a long track-record of fulfillment. They have natural body care aromatherapy, flower essences, crystals and tumbled stones, homeopathy, herbal products, vitamins and supplements, videos, books, audio tapes, candles, incense and bulk herbs, teas, massage tools and products and numerous alternative health items across a wide range of categories.

WHOLESALE:

Wholesale suppliers sell to stores and practitioners, not to individual consumers buying for their own personal use. Individual consumers should contact the RETAIL supplier listed below. Wholesale accounts should contact with business name, resale number or practitioner license in order to obtain a wholesale catalog and set up an account.

Lotus Light Enterprises, Inc.

P O Box 1008 3G
Silver Lake, WI 53170 USA
414 889 8501 (phone)
414 889 8591 (fax)
800 548 3824 (toll free order line)

RETAIL:

Retail suppliers provide products by mail order direct to consumers for their personal use. Stores or practitioners should contact the wholesale supplier listed above.

Internatural

33719 116th Street 3G
Twin Lakes, WI 53181 USA
800 643 4221 (toll free order line)
414 889 8581 office phone
WEB SITE: www.internatural.com

Web site includes an extensive annotated catalog of more than 7000 products that can be ordered "on line" for your convenience 24 hours a day, 7 days a week.